# Eating Well with Diabetes

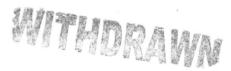

By Jane Finsand,
Edith White, M.Ed.,
Karin Cadwell, Ph.D., R.N.

Sterling Publishing Co., Inc.
New York

10  9  8  7  6  5  4  3  2  1

Published by Sterling Publishing Co., Inc.
387 Park Avenue South, New York, NY 10016
This book is comprised of material from the following Sterling titles:
*The Complete Diabetic Cookbook* © 1987 by Sterling Publishing Co., Inc.
*Great Diabetic Desserts & Sweets* © 1995 by Karin Cadwell and Edith White
*Diabetic Candy, Cookie & Dessert Cookbook* © 1982 by Mary Jane Finsand

© 2002 by Sterling Publishing Co., Inc.
Distributed in Canada by Sterling Publishing
c/o Canadian Manda Group, One Atlantic Avenue, Suite 105
Toronto, Ontario, Canada M6K 3E7
Distributed in Great Britain by Chrysalis Books Group PLC
The Chrysalis Building, Bramley Road, London W10 6SP, England
Distributed in Australia by Capricorn Link (Australia) Pty. Ltd.
P.O. Box 704, Windsor, NSW 2756, Australia

Manufactured in the United States of America

ISBN 1-4027-1719-9

# Contents

# Introduction

*Eating Well with Diabetes* was created to help beginning as well as more experienced cooks by adding to their repertoire of diabetic recipes. No one wants to think of him or herself as being on a restricted diet, yet all of us are on a diet; therefore, it is the word "restricted" which must be removed. This cookbook is designed to remove the word "restricted," to give a more tasteful and varied food intake for everyone. It is meant to reduce and simplify the day-to-day preparation of healthful, good food. There are no complete menus, but rather, individual recipes that will open up new cooking horizons. By using the simple exchange or caloric values, anyone can whip up a gourmet meal with no fear of overindulgence.

If you look at the number of savory and sweet recipes, you will notice that the dessert section is nearly a large as the rest of the book. This reflects the fact that there are so many people with a sweet tooth, and many or more who do not feel a meal is complete without dessert.

Eating a piece of pie or candy bar without knowing the exchange value or calorie count can be disastrous to any diet. All of us should be aware of our total calorie intake and compare it to our total calorie output daily. To make weight reduction or a healthy diet as pleasant as possible, it is important to realize that eating can still be made an enjoyable experience.

It would be an overstatement to suggest that this cookbook has all the answers to feeding a diabetic. It does not. However, I hope that *Eating Well with Diabetes* will help family cooks form everyday good eating habits for the diabetic and for the rest of the family as well.

# Using the Recipes for Your Diet

All recipes have been developed using diet substitutions for sugar, syrup, sauces, toppings, puddings, gelatins, mayonnaise, salad dressings, and imitation or lo-cal dairy and non-dairy products.

Remember, diet is the key word for controlling diabetes, and each person's diet is prescribed individually by a doctor or counselor who has been trained to mold your daily life to your diet requirements. DO NOT try to outguess them. If you have any questions about any diabetic recipes, ask your diet counselor.

Read the recipes carefully, then assemble all equipment and ingredients. "Added Touch" ingredients are flavorful additions, but not necessary to the recipe's success. Substitutions or additions of herbs and spices or flavorings to a recipe may be made by using the guide for Spices and Herbs, or for Flavorings and Extracts; they will make any of the recipes distinctively your own.

Use standard measuring equipment (whether metric or customary), and be sure to measure accurately. Remember, these recipes are good for everyone, not just the diabetic.

**CUSTOMARY TERMS**

| | |
|---|---|
| t. | teaspoon |
| T. | tablespoon |
| c. | cup |
| pkg. | package |
| pt. | pint |
| qt. | quart |
| oz. | ounce |
| lb. | pound |
| F | Fahrenheit |
| in. | inch |

**METRIC SYMBOLS**

| | |
|---|---|
| mL | milliliter |
| L | liter |
| g | gram |
| kg | kilogram |
| mm | millimeter |
| cm | centimeter |
| C | Celsius |

# GUIDE TO APPROXIMATE EQUIVALENTS

| Customary: | | | | Metric: | |
|---|---|---|---|---|---|
| ounces; | | | | | grams; |
| pounds | cups | tablespoons | teaspoons | millilitres | killograms |
| | | | ¼ t. | 1 mL | |
| | | | ½ t. | 2 mL | |
| | | | 1 t. | 5 mL | |
| | | | 2 t. | 10 mL | |
| ½ oz. | | 1 T. | 3 t. | 15 mL | 15 g |
| 1 oz. | | 2 T. | 6 t. | 30 mL | 30 g |
| 2 oz. | ¼ c. | 4 T. | 12 t. | 60 mL | |
| 4 oz. | ½ c. | 8 T. | 24 t. | 125 mL | |
| 8 oz. | 1 c. | 16 T. | 48 t. | 250 mL | |
| 2.2 lb. | | | | | 1 kg |

Keep in mind that this is not an exact conversion, but generally may be used for food measurement.

# GUIDE TO PAN SIZES
## Baking Pans

| Customary: | Metric: | Holds: |
|---|---|---|
| 8-inch pie | 20-cm pie | 600 mL |
| 9-inch pie | 23-cm pie | 1 L |
| 10-inch pie | 25-cm pie | 1.3 L |
| 8-inch round | 20-cm round | 1 L |
| 9-inch round | 23-cm round | 1.5 L |
| 8-inch square | 20-cm square | 2 L |
| 9-inch square | 23-cm square | 2.5 L |
| 9 x 5 x 2-inch loaf | 23 x 13 x 5-cm loaf | 2 L |
| 9-inch tube | 23-cm tube | 3 L |
| 10-inch tube | 25-cm tube | 3 L |
| 13 x 9 x 2-inch | 33 x 23 x 5-cm | 3.5L |
| 14 x 10-inch cookie tin | 35 x 25-cm cookie tin | |
| 15 ½ x 10 ½ x 1-inch jelly-roll | 39 x 25 x 3-cm jelly-roll | |

## Cooking Pans and Casseroles

| Customary: | Metric: |
| --- | --- |
| 1 quart | 1 L |
| 2 quart | 2 L |
| 3 quart | 3 L |

## OVEN COOKING GUIDES

Follow this guide for oven temperature:

| Fahrenheit °F | Oven heat | Celsius °C |
| --- | --- | --- |
| 250-275° | very slow | 120-135° |
| 300-325° | slow | 150-165° |
| 350-375° | moderate | 177-190° |
| 400-425° | hot | 200-220° |
| 450-475° | very hot | 230-245° |
| 475-500° | hottest | 250-290° |

Use this meat thermometer probe guide to check the meat's internal temperature:

| Fahrenheit °F | Desired Doneness | | Celsius °C |
| --- | --- | --- | --- |
| 140° | Beef: | rare | 60° |
| 150° | | medium | 65° |
| 170° | | well done | 75° |
| 160° | Lamb: | medium | 70° |
| 170° | | well done | 75° |
| 180° | Veal: | well done | 80° |
| 180° | Pork: | well done | 80° |
| 185° | Poultry: | well done | 85° |

# SPICES AND HERBS

*Allspice:*  Cinnamon, ginger, nutmeg flavor; used in breads, pastries, jellies, jams, pickles.

*Anise:*  Licorice flavor; used in candies, breads, fruit, wine, liqueurs.

*Basil:*  Sweet-strong flavor; used in meat, cheese, egg, tomato dishes.

*Bay Leaf:*  Sweet flavor; used in meat, fish, vegetable dishes.

*Celery:*  Unique, pleasantly bitter flavor; used in anything not sweet.

*Chive:*  Light onion flavor; used in anything where onion should be delicate.

*Chili Powder:*  Hot, pungent flavor; used in Mexican, Spanish dishes.

*Cinnamon:*  Pungent, sweet flavor; used in pastries, breads, pickles, wine, beer, liqueurs.

*Clove:*  Pungent, sweet flavor; used for ham, sauces, pastries, puddings, fruit, wine, liqueurs.

*Coriander:*  Butter-lemon flavor; used for pork, cookies, cakes, pies, puddings, fruit, wine and liqueur punches.

*Garlic:*  Strong, aromatic flavor; used in Italian, French, and many meat dishes.

*Ginger:* Strong, pungent flavor; used in anything sweet, plus with beer, brandy, liqueurs.

*Marjoram:* Sweet, semi-pungent flavor; used in poultry, lamb, egg, vegetable dishes.

*Nutmeg:* Sweet, nutty flavor; used in pastries, puddings, vegetables.

*Oregano:* Sweet, pungent flavor; used in meat, pasta, vegetable dishes.

*Paprika:* Light, sweet flavor; used in salads, vegetables, poultry, fish, egg dishes; often used to brighten bland-colored casseroles or entrées.

*Rosemary:* Fresh, sweet flavor; used in soups, meat and vegetable dishes.

*Sage:* Pungent, bitter flavor; used in stuffings, sausages, some cheese dishes.

*Thyme:* Pungent, semi-bitter flavor; used in salty dishes or soups.

*Woodruff:* Sweet vanilla flavor; used in wines, punches.

**Note:** Metric equivalents for the stronger spices and herbs vary for each recipe to allow for individual effectiveness at convenient measurements.

# FLAVORINGS AND EXTRACTS

Orange, lime, and lemon peel give vegetables, pastries, and puddings a fresh, clean flavor; liqueur flavors, such as brandy or rum, give cakes and other desserts a company flare. Choose from the following to add some zip without calories:

| | | |
|---|---|---|
| Almond | Butter Rum | Pecan |
| Anise (Licorice) | Cherry | Peppermint |
| Apricot | Clove | Pineapple |
| Banana Crème | Coconut | Raspberry |
| Blackberry | Grape | Rum |
| Black Walnut | Hazelnut | Sassafras |
| Blueberry | Lemon | Sherry |
| Brandy | Lime | Strawberry |
| Burnt Sugar | Mint | Vanilla |
| Butter | Orange | Walnut |
| Butternut | | |

# APPETIZERS

## Fruit Dip

| | | |
|---|---|---|
| 8 ounces | plain lo-cal yogurt | 240 g |
| 4 tablespoons | lo-cal preserves | 60 mL |
| ½ teaspoon | ground allspice | 2 mL |
| ½ teaspoon | lemon juice | 2 mL |

Combine all ingredients. Whip until fluffy. Chill thoroughly.

**YIELD:** 1 cup (250 mL)
**EXCHANGE:** 1 milk
**CALORIES:** 192

## Onion Dip

| | | |
|---|---|---|
| 4 ounces | plan lo-cal yogurt | 120 g |
| ¼ cup | onions (finely chopped) | 60 mL |
| 1 teaspoon | lemon juice | 5 mL |
| 1 tablespoon | parsley | 15 mL |
| Dash each | hot pepper sauce, horseradish, salt, pepper | dash each |

Combine all ingredients. Chill thoroughly.

**YIELD:** ¾ cup (190 mL)
**EXCHANGE:** ½ milk
½ vegetable
**CALORIES:** 72

# Shrimp Dip

| | | |
|---|---|---|
| 5 small | shrimp | 5 small |
| ½ teaspoon | Worcestershire sauce | 2 mL |
| 1 teaspoon | lemon juice | 5 mL |
| 4 ounces | plain lo-cal yogurt | 120 g |
| ¼ cup | Chili Sauce (page 129) | 60 mL |

Crush shrimp. Sprinkle with Worcestershire sauce and lemon juice. Combine yogurt and Chili Sauce. Add crushed shrimp; stir to blend. Chill.

**YIELD:** ¾ cup (190 mL)
**EXCHANGE:** 1 meat
½ milk
½ fruit
**CALORIES:** 108

# Avocado Crisps

| | | |
|---|---|---|
| 1 | very ripe avocado | 1 |
| 1 teaspoon | lemon juice | 5 mL |
| 1 teaspoon | grated onion | 5 mL |
| 1 teaspoon | onion salt | 5 mL |
| 1 teaspoon | paprika | 5 mL |
| ½ teaspoon | marjoram | 2 mL |
| | thin crackers | |

Peel and mash avocado. Add remaining ingredients. Beat until smooth. Spread thinly on crackers.

**YIELD:** 45 servings
**EXCHANGE 5 SERVINGS:** 1 bread
1 fat
**CALORIES 5 SERVINGS:** 108

# Stuffed Celery

| | | |
|---|---|---|
| 2 5-inch | stalks celery | 2 12-cm |
| 1 tablespoon | cream cheese (softened) | 30 mL |
| ¼ teaspoon | onion powder | 1 mL |
| dash | paprika | dash |
| | salt and pepper to taste | |

Thoroughly rinse and drain celery. Combine cream cheese, onion powder, and paprika. Blend until smooth and creamy. Add salt and pepper. Fill celery stalks. Chill.

**YIELD:** 1 serving
**EXCHANGE:** 1 fat
**CALORIES:** 50

# Cheese Appetizers

| | | |
|---|---|---|
| 4 ounces | cheddar cheese (shredded) | 120 g |
| 2 tablespoons | margarine | 30 mL |
| ½ cup | flour | 125 mL |
| 1 teaspoon | onion (grated) | 5 mL |
| ½ teaspoon | salt | 2 mL |
| ¼ teaspoon | pepper | 1 mL |

Blend cheese and margarine until smooth. Add flour, onion, salt, and pepper. Stir until smooth. Shape dough into a roll, 1¼ inch (3.5 cm) in diameter. Wrap in plastic wrap or aluminum foil. Chill. Cut into ¼-inch (6-mm) slices. Bake at 400° F (200° C) for 8 minutes.

**YIELD:** 24 servings
**EXCHANGE 1 SERVING:** ½ fat
¼ bread
**CALORIES 1 SERVING:** 37

# Cucumbers in Yogurt

| | | |
|---|---|---|
| 1 | cucumber | 1 |
| 1 small | onion | 1 small |
| 1 teaspoon | salt | 5 mL |
| ½ teaspoon | garlic powder | 2 mL |
| 1 teaspoon | lemon juice | 5 mL |
| ½ teaspoon | marjoram | 2 mL |
| 8 ounces | lo-cal yogurt | 240 g |

Peel and thinly slice cucumber and onion. Sprinkle with salt. Allow to rest 15 minutes. Drain and pat dry. Combine garlic powder, lemon juice, marjoram, and yogurt; mix thoroughly. Fold in sliced cucumber and onion. Chill.

**YIELD:** 2 cups (500 mL)
**EXCHANGE:** 1 milk
**CALORIES:** 100

# Summer Chicken Canapés

| | | |
|---|---|---|
| 4 ounces | ground cooked chicken | 120 g |
| 2 tablespoons | margarine (softened) | 30 mL |
| ¼ teaspoon | dry mustard | 2 mL |
| ½ teaspoon | meat tenderizer | 2 mL |
| ½ teaspoon | salt | 2 mL |
| ⅛ teaspoon | pepper | 1 mL |
| ⅛-inch thick | cucumber slices | 6-mm thick |

Combine chicken, margarine, dry mustard, meat tenderizer, salt, and pepper. Mix thoroughly. Chill. To make canapé: Place 1 teaspoon (5 mL) of chicken mixture in center of cucumber slice.

**YIELD:** 24 servings
**EXCHANGE 2 SERVINGS:** ½ fat
**CALORIES 2 SERVINGS:** 28

# Garlic Bites

| | | |
|---|---|---|
| 1 slice | white bread | 1 slice |
| 2 teaspoons | lo-cal margarine | 10 mL |
| ¼ teaspoon | garlic powder | 2 mL |

Remove crust from bread; cut bread into ¼-inch (6-mm) cubes. Melt margarine in small pan. Add garlic powder and heat until sizzling. Add bread cubes; sauté, tossing frequently until brown. Drain and cool.

**YIELD:** 2 servings
**EXCHANGE 1 SERVING:** ½ bread
1 fat
**CALORIES 1 SERVING:** 79

# Liver Paste

| | |
|---|---|
| 3 ounces chicken livers | 90 g |
| 1 tablespoon onion (finely chopped) | 15 mL |
| 1 egg (hard cooked) | 1 |
| 2 teaspoons margarine | 10 mL |
| 1 tablespoon evaporated (regular or skim) milk | 15 mL |
| Salt and pepper to taste | |

Boil chicken livers and onion in small amount of water until tender. Drain. Finely chop the egg. Mash livers, onion, egg, and margarine until well blended. Add milk; blend thoroughly. Add salt and pepper.

**YIELD:** 24 servings, 1 teaspoon (5mL) each
**EXCHANGE 3 SERVINGS:** ½ medium-fat meat
**CALORIES 3 SERVINGS:** 39

# Hors d'Oeuvre Spreads

**YIELD:** ¼ cup (60 mL) spread for 24 crackers or ½ teaspoon (3 mL) per cracker.
**EXCHANGE PER SERVING:** ½ fat plus cracker exchange
Use one of the following as a spread for 24 small crackers:

## ANCHOVY

| 1 ounce | anchovy fillets | 30 g |
| ¼ cup | lo-cal margarine | 60 mL |

Rinse fillets in cold water; pat dry. Grind or chop fine; blend with margarine. Allow to rest.

**EXCHANGE ¼ CUP (60 mL):** 12 fat
1 meat
**CALORIES ¼ CUP (60 mL):** 250

## CAVIAR

| 2 tablespoons | caviar | 30 mL |
| ¼ cup | lo-cal margarine | 60 mL |

Combine caviar and margarine. Refrigerate overnight.

**EXCHANGE ¼ CUP (60 mL):** 12 fat
1 meat
**CALORIES ¼ CUP (60 mL):** 280

## CRABMEAT

| 2 tablespoons | crabmeat | 30 mL |
| ¼ cup | lo-cal margarine | 60 mL |

Crush crabmeat; blend with margarine. Refrigerate overnight.

**EXCHANGE ¼ CUP (60 mL):** 12 fat
½ meat
**CALORIES ¼ CUP (60 mL):** 230

## GARLIC

| ¼ teaspoon | garlic | 2 mL |
| dash | salt | dash |
| ¼ cup | lo-cal margarine | 60 mL |

Blend ingredients together.

**EXCHANGE ¼ CUP (60 ML):** 12 fat
**CALORIES ¼ CUP (60 ML):** 200

## HERB

| Dash each | marjoram, oregano, onion (chopped), salt, pepper | dash each |
| ¼ cup | lo-cal margarine | 60 mL |

Blend ingredients together; allow to rest at room temperature 2 hours.

**EXCHANGE ¼ CUP (60 ML):** 12 fat
**CALORIES ¼ CUP (60 ML):** 200

## HORSERADISH

| 1 tablespoon | horseradish (grated) | 15 mL |
| 1 teaspoon | parsley (chopped) | 5 mL |
| ¼ cup | lo-cal margarine | 60 mL |

Blend ingredients together; refrigerate overnight.

**EXCHANGE ¼ CUP (60 ML):** 12 fat
**CALORIES ¼ CUP (60 ML):** 200

## LEMON

| 1 teaspoon | lemon juice | 5 mL |
| dash | salt | dash |
| ¼ teaspoon | parsley | 2 mL |
| ¼ cup | loc-cal margarine | 60 mL |

Blend ingredients together.

**EXCHANGE ¼ CUP (60 mL):** 12 fat
**CALORIES ¼ CUP (60 mL):** 200

## MUSTARD

| | | |
|---|---|---|
| 2 teaspoons | Dijon mustard | 10 mL |
| ¼ cup | margarine | 60 mL |

Blend ingredients together.

**EXCHANGE ¼ CUP (60 mL):** 12 fat
**CALORIES ¼ CUP (60 mL):** 200

*Note:* Exchange and caloric figures above do not include crackers.

Spreads may be topped with 1 teaspoon (5 mL):

| | | |
|---|---|---|
| Chicken | Salami | Crabmeat |
| Chicken liver | Sausage | Lobster |
| Ham | Tuna | |

**EXCHANGE TO ADD 6 CRACKERS:** 1 meat
plus cracker exchange

Bacon     Avocodo

**EXCHANGE TO ADD 5 CRACKERS:** 1 fat
plus cracker exchange

| | | |
|---|---|---|
| Cauliflower | Mushrooms | Green pepper |
| Celery | Onion | Radish |
| Cucumber | Parsley | Tomato flesh |

**EXCHANGE:** Only cracker exchange

# Smoke Salmon Canapés

| 8 ounces | smoked salmon | 240 g |
| 3 ounces | cream cheese | 90 g |
| ½ teaspoon | lemon juice | 2 mL |
| 1 teaspoon | milk | 5 mL |
| dash each | thyme, sage, salt, pepper | dash each |

Place smoked salmon in blender. Blend until fine. Combine cream cheese, lemon juice, and milk. Stir to make a paste. Add seasonings. Mix well. Add salmon; blend thoroughly. Roll into 22 balls. Chill.

**YIELD:** 22 servings
**EXCHANGE 2 SERVINGS:** 1 meat
**CALORIES 2 SERVINGS:** 68

# Swiss Morsels

| 8 ounces | Swiss cheese (grated) | 240 g |
| 4 ounces | ham (grated) | 120 g |
| 2 tablespoons | margarine (softened) | 30 mL |
| ¼ teaspoon | thyme | 1 mL |

Combine all ingredients; mix thoroughly. Shape 2 teaspoons (10 mL) of mixture into a ball. Repeat with remaining mixture.

**YIELD:** 34 servings
**EXCHANGE 1 SERVING:** ½ high-fat meat
**CALORIES 1 SERVING:** 51

# SOUPS AND STEWS

## Chicken Broth

| | | |
|---|---|---|
| 2 pound | hen (cut up) | 1 kg |
| ½ medium stalk | celery (chopped) | ½ medium |
| 8 to 10 | green onions (chopped) | 8 to 10 |
| 2 tablespoons | parsley (chopped) | 30 mL |
| 2 teaspoons | salt | 10 mL |
| 1 teaspoon | thyme | 5 mL |
| 1 teaspoon | marjoram | 5 mL |
| ½ teaspoon | pepper | 2 mL |

Wash chicken pieces; place in large kettle. Cover with 2 quarts (2 L) water; bring to a boil, cover and cook 1 hour or until chicken is tender. Add remaining ingredients; simmer 1 hour. Remove chicken; strain broth. Refrigerate broth overnight. Remove all fat from surface before reheating broth.

**YIELD:**     2 quarts (2 L) broth
**EXCHANGE:**  Negligible
**CALORIES:**  Negligible

# Beef Broth

| | | |
|---|---|---|
| 3 to 4 pounds | beef soup bones or chuck roast | 1½ to 2 kg |
| ½ stalk | celery (chopped) | ½ stalk |
| 3 | carrots (sliced) | 3 |
| 1 | medium onion (chopped) | 1 medium |
| ½ | green pepper (chopped) | ½ |
| 2 | bay leaves | 2 |
| ½ t. each | thyme, marjoram, paprika, pepper | 2 mL each |
| 2 t. | salt | 10 mL |

Place beef in large kettle; cover with 2 quarts (2 L) water. Bring to a boil, cover and cook 2 hours, or until meat is tender. Add remaining ingredients; simmer 1 hour. Remove beef; strain broth. Refrigerate broth overnight. Remove all fat from surface before reheating broth.

**YIELD:**  2 quarts (2 L) broth
**EXCHANGE:**  Negligible
**CALORIES:**  Negligible

# Broth with Vegetables

Cook ½ cup (125 mL) vegetables or combination of vegetables in boiling salted water; drain. Add to hot broth just before serving.

**MICROWAVE:** Add ½ cup (125 mL) vegetables (no water needed). Cook on High for 3 minutes. Add to hot broth just before serving.

**YIELD:**       ½ cup (125 mL)
**EXCHANGE:**  ½ vegetable
**CALORIES:**   18

# Broth with Noodles

Cook ¼ cup (60 mL) noodles or broken spaghetti in boiling salted water; drain. Add to hot broth just before serving.

**MICROWAVE:** Add ¼ cup (60 mL) noodles or pasta to 2 cups (500 mL) boiling salted water. Cook on High for 3 minutes. Hold 3 minutes. Drain. Add to hot broth just before serving.

**YIELD:** ½ cup (125 mL)
**EXCHANGE:** 1 bread
**CALORIES:** 68

# Broth Italiano

| ⅛ cup | vermicelli (broken) | 30 mL |
|---|---|---|
| 1 cup | broth | 250 mL |
| 1 ounce | thinly sliced prosciutto (shredded) | 30 g |
| ⅛ teaspoon | garlic powder | 1 mL |
| ⅛ teaspoon | marjoram | 1 mL |
| 1 tablespoon | Parmesan cheese (grated) | 15 mL |

Cook vermicelli in boiling salted water; drain and rinse. Bring broth to a boil. Add proscuitto, garlic powder, and marjoram. Simmer 5 minutes. Add vermicelli. Pour into bowl. Sprinkle Parmesan cheese over top.

**YIELD:** 1¼ cups (310 mL)
**EXCHANGE:** ½ bread
1 medium-fat meat
**CALORIES:** 107

# Broth Madeira

Add 1 tablespoon (15 mL) Madeira to 1 cups (250 mL) broth. Bring just to a boil. Garnish with lemon slice and fresh chopped parsley.

**MICROWAVE:** Add 1 tablespoon (15 mL) Madeira to 1 cup (250 mL) broth. Cook on High for 2 minutes. garnish with lemon slice and fresh chopped parsley.

**YIELD:**  1 cup (250 mL)
**EXCHANGE:** Negligible
**CALORIES:** Negligible

# Vegetable Broth

| 1 cup | onion (chopped) | 250 mL |
|---|---|---|
| 2 cups | carrots (diced) | 500 mL |
| 1 cup | celery (chopped) | 250 mL |
| 2 cups | spinach (cut in small pieces) | 500 mL |
| 2 cups | tomato (peeled and chopped) | 500 mL |
| 1 | bay leaf | 1 |
| 2 tablespoons | parsley or parsley flakes | 30 mL |
| ½ teaspoon | thyme | 3 mL |
| 1 blade | mace | 1 blade |
| ¼ teaspoon | garlic or garlic powder | 1 mL |
| 1 tablespoon | Worcestershire | 15 mL |
| | salt to taste | |

Place vegetables in large kettle. Cover with 2 to 3 quarts (2 to 3 L) water. Bring to a boil; reduce heat and simmer for 2 hours. Stir frequently. Add seasonings. Simmer 1 hour. Strain. Add water to make 2 quarts (2 L).

**YIELD:**  2 quarts (2 L) broth
**EXCHANGE:** Negligible
**CALORIES:** Negligible

# Broth Orientale

| | | |
|---|---|---|
| 2 tablespoons | rice | 30 mL |
| 1 ½ cups | vegetable broth | 375 mL |
| 1 tablespoon | celery (thinly sliced) | 15 mL |
| ½ teaspoon | onion (finely chopped) | 3 mL |
| 1 tablespoon | bean sprouts | 15 mL |
| 1 | water chestnut (thinly sliced) | 1 |
| | salt to taste | |

Add rice to cold vegetable broth; bring to boil. Reduce heat; simmer 20 minutes. Add celery, onion, bean sprouts and water chestnut; simmer 10 minutes. Add salt.

**MICROWAVE:** Add rice to cold broth; heat to a boil. Cover. Hold 15 minutes. Add remaining ingredients, except salt. Cook 3 minutes. Hold 5 minutes. Add salt.

**YIELD:** 1 ¼ cups (310 mL)
**EXCHANGE:** ¹/₈ bread
¹/₈ vegetable
**CALORIES:** 11

# Tomato Beef Bouillon

| | | |
|---|---|---|
| 2 tablespoons | margarine | 30 mL |
| ¼ cup | onion (chopped) | 60 mL |
| 46 ounces | tomato juice | 1½ L |
| 2 cans | beef broth or | 2 cans |
| 2½ cups | homemade beef broth | 625 mL |
| 1 | bay leaf | 1 |
| 1 teaspoon | salt | 5 mL |
| ½ teaspoon | pepper | 2 mL |

Heat margarine in a large saucepan. Add onion and cook until tender. Add tomato juice, beef broth (canned or home-made), bay leaf, salt, and pepper; heat thoroughly. DO NOT BOIL. Remove bay leaf. Ladle into warm bowls.

*Added Touch:* Top each serving with 1 teaspoon (5 mL) grated American cheese.

**YIELD:**                        8 servings, 1 cup (250 mL) each
**EXCHANGE 1 SERVING:** ¼ vegetable
                                 1 fat
**CALORIES 1 SERVING:**     58

# Greek Egg Lemon Soup

| 2 quarts | chicken broth | 2 L |
| 3 | eggs (separated) | 3 |
|  | Juice of 1 lemon |  |

Bring broth to a boil in saucepan. Beat egg whites until stiff. Add egg yolks. Beat slowly until mixture is a light yellow. Add lemon juice gradually, beating constantly. Pour small amount of chicken broth into egg mixture. Pour egg mixture into hot broth, beating constantly.

**YIELD:**                        8 servings, 1 cup (250 mL) each
**EXCHANGE 1 SERVING:** ¼ high-fat meat
**CALORIES 1 SERVING:**     27

# Quick Egg Soup

| | | |
|---|---|---|
| 1½ cups | boiling water | 375 mL |
| 1 cube | vegetable bouillon | 1 cube |
| 1 | egg | 1 |

Dissolve bouillon cube in boiling water; remove from heat. Beat egg; blend into vegetable broth. Reheat slowly. DO NOT BOIL.

**YIELD:** 1½ cups (375 mL)
**EXCHANGE:** 1 medium-fat meat
**CALORIES:** 80

# German Cabbage Soup

| | | |
|---|---|---|
| 2 ounces | ground beef round | 60 g |
| 2 tablespoons | onion (grated) | 30 mL |
| dash each | mustard, soy sauce, salt, pepper | dash each |
| 1 tablespoon | dry red wine | 15 mL |
| 1¼ cups | beef broth | 300 mL |
| 2 large | cabbage leaves (cut in pieces) | 2 large |
| ½ medium | tomato (cubed) | ½ medium |
| ½ teaspoon | fresh parsley (chopped) | 2 mL |

Combine ground round, onion, mustard, soy sauce, salt, and pepper; mix thoroughly. Form into tiny meatballs. Add wine to broth; bring to a boil. Add meatballs to broth, one at a time. Bring to boil again. Cook meatballs 5 minutes; remove to soup bowl. Add cabbage and tomatoes to broth. Simmer 5 minutes. Pour over meatballs. Garnish with parsley.

**YIELD:** 1½ cups (375 mL)
**EXCHANGE:** 1 medium-fat meat
½ vegetable
**CALORIES:** 55

# Borscht

| | | |
|---|---|---|
| 16-ounce can | beets with juice | 500-g can |
| 2 tablespoons | sugar replacement | 30 mL |
| ¾ teaspoon | salt | 3 mL |
| 3 tablespoons | lemon juice | 45 mL |
| ½ teaspoon | thyme | 2 mL |
| 1 | egg (well beaten) | 1 |

Purée beats in blender. Add enough water to make 1 quart (1 L). Pour into saucepan. Add sugar replacement, salt, lemon juice, and thyme; heat to a boil. Remove from heat. Add small amount of hot beet mixture to egg. Stir egg mixture into beet mixture. Return to heat; cook and stir until hot. DO NOT BOIL.

**YIELD:** 4 servings, 1 cup (250 mL) each
**EXCHANGE 1 SERVING:** 1 bread
¼ high-fat meat
**CALORIES 1 SERVING:** 104
*Added Touch:* Top each serving with 1 teaspoon (5 mL) lo-cal sour cream.

# French Meatball Soup

| | | |
|---|---|---|
| 2 tablespoons | rice (uncooked) | 30 mL |
| 2 ounces | ground beef round | 60 g |
| 1 tablespoon | egg (raw, beaten) | 15 mL |
| 1 teaspoon | onion (grated) | 5 mL |
| dash each | garlic, parsley, nutmeg | dash each |
| 2 tablespoons | dry red wine | 30 mL |
| 1¼ cups | beef broth | 300 mL |
| | salt and pepper to taste | |

Add rice to 1 cup (250 mL) salted water. Boil 5 minutes; drain well. Blend rice, ground round, egg, onion, garlic, parsley, and nutmeg; form into small meatballs. Add wine to broth; bring to a boil. Drop meatballs into hot broth, one at a time. Bring to boil again; reduce heat. Simmer 20 minutes. Add salt and pepper.

**MICROWAVE:** Add rice to 1 cup (250 mL) salted water. Bring to a boil. Hold 5 minutes; drain well. Combine meatball ingredients as above. Bring wine and broth to a boil. Drop meatballs into hot broth, one at a time. Bring to a boil again. Set aside 10 minutes. Add salt and pepper.

**YIELD:** 1½ cups (375 mL)
**EXCHANGE:** 1 medium-fat meat
½ bread
**CALORIES:** 71

# Ham and Split Pea soup

| 2 pounds | meaty ham bone | 1 kg |
| 1 | bay leaf 1 | |
| 2 cups | dried green split peas, soaked overnight | 500 mL |
| 1 cup | onions (chopped) | 250 mL |
| 1 cup | celery (cubed) | 250 mL |
| 1 cup | carrots (grated) | 250 mL |
| | salt and pepper to taste | |

Cover ham bone and bay leaf with water. Simmer for 2 to 2½ hours. Remove bone and strain liquid. Refrigerate overnight. Remove lean meat from bone; set aside. Remove fat from surface of liquid. Heat liquid; add enough water to make 2½ quarts (2½ L). Add peas; simmer for 20 minutes. Remove from heat and allow to stand 1 hour. Add onions, celery, carrots, and lean pieces of ham. Add salt and pepper. Simmer for 40 minutes. Stir occasionally.

**YIELD:** 10 servings
**EXCHANGE 1 SERVING:** ½ high-fat meat
1 vegetable
**CALORIES 1 SERVING:** 204

# Cream of Chicken and Almond Soup

| | | |
|---|---|---|
| 1 cup | chicken broth | 250 mL |
| 1 | whole clove | 1 |
| 1 sprig | parsley | 1 sprig |
| ½ | bay leaf | ½ |
| pinch | mace | pinch |
| 1 tablespoon | celery (sliced) | 15 mL |
| 1 tablespoon | carrot (diced) | 15 mL |
| 1 teaspoon | onion (diced) | 5 mL |
| 2 teaspoons | stale bread crumbs | 10 mL |
| ½ ounce | chicken breast (cubed) | 15 g |
| 1 teaspoon | blanched almonds (crushed) | 5 mL |
| ¼ cup | skim milk | 60 mL |
| 1 teaspoon | flour | 5 mL |
| | salt and pepper to taste | |

Heat chicken broth, clove, parsley, bay leaf, and mace to a boil; remove from heat. Allow to rest 10 minutes; strain. Add celery, carrot, onion, bread crumbs, chicken, and almonds to seasoned chicken broth; simmer 20 minutes. Blend in skim milk and flour. Remove soup from heat; add milk mixture. Return to heat. Simmer (do not boil) 3 to 5minutes. Add salt and pepper.

**YIELD:** 1½ cups (375 mL)
**EXCHANGE:** ½ lean meat
1 vegetable
¼ milk
**CALORIES:** 89

# Crab Chowder

| | | |
|---|---|---|
| 1 cup | milk | 250 mL |
| 1 teaspoon | flour | 5 mL |
| ¼ cup | water | 60 mL |
| ¼ cup | cooked crabmeat (flaked) | 60 mL |
| 3 tablespoons | mushroom pieces | 45 mL |
| 3 tablespoons | asparagus pieces | 45 mL |
| | salt and pepper to taste | |

Blend milk, flour, and water thoroughly; pour into saucepan. Add crabmeat, mushrooms, and asparagus. Cook over low heat until slightly thickened. Add salt and pepper.

**YIELD:** 1 cup (250 mL)
**EXCHANGE:** 1 milk
1 vegetable
1 lean meat
**CALORIES:** 150

# Clam Chowder

| | | |
|---|---|---|
| 1 slice | bacon | 1 slice |
| 1½ cups | fish or vegetable broth | 375 mL |
| 2 tablespoons | carrot (diced) | 30 mL |
| 1 tablespoon | onion (diced) | 15 mL |
| 1 tablespoon | celery (diced) | 15 mL |
| 1 large | tomato (diced) | 1 large |
| 1 medium | potato (diced) | 1 medium |
| dash each | thyme, rosemary, salt, pepper | dash each |
| 1 teaspoon | flour | 5 mL |
| ¼ cup | water | 60 mL |
| 1 ounce | clams | 30 g |

Cook bacon until crisp; drain and crumble. Combine broth, carrot, onion, celery, tomato, potato, and seasonings. Simmer until vegetables are tender. Blend flour and water;

stir into chowder. Reduce heat. Add clams and crumbled bacon. Heat to thicken slightly.

**MICROWAVE:** Combine vegetables with broth and seasonings; cover. Cook on High for 4 minutes, or until vegetables are tender. Add flour-water mixture. Cook 30 seconds; stir. Add clams and bacon; stir. Cook 30 seconds. Hold 3 minutes.

**YIELD:**     2 cups (500 mL)
**EXCHANGE:**  1 lean meat
               1 fat
               1 vegetable
               1 bread
**CALORIES:**  200

# Fish Chowder

| | | |
|---|---|---|
| 2 cups | water | 500 mL |
| 3 ounces | bullhead fillet | 90 g |
| 1 medium | potato (diced) | 1 medium |
| 3 tablespoons | onion (diced) | 45 mL |
| 3 tablespoons | celery (diced) | 45 mL |
| 2 tablespoons | carrot (Diced) | 30 mL |
| 1 medium | tomato (diced) | 1 medium |
| | Salt and pepper to taste | |

Combine all ingredients in saucepan. Heat to a boil; cover and reduce heat. Simmer 1 to 1½ hours.

**YIELD:**                    3 servings, 1 cup (250 mL) each
**EXCHANGE 1 SERVING:**       1 medium-fat meat
                              ½ vegetable
                              ½ bread
**CALORIES 1 SERVING:**       81

# Oyster Stew

| | | |
|---|---|---|
| 1 teaspoon | flour | 5 mL |
| 1 tablespoon | celery (minced) | 15 mL |
| 1 teaspoon | salt | 5 mL |
| dash each | Worcestershire sauce, soy sauce | dash each |
| 1 tablespoon | water | 15 mL |
| 1 ounce | oysters (with liquid) | 30 g |
| 1 teaspoon | butter | 5 mL |
| 1 cup | skim milk | 250 mL |

Blend flour, celery, seasoning, and water in saucepan; add oysters with liquid, and butter. Simmer over low heat until edges of oysters curl. Remove from heat; add skim milk. Reheat over low heat. Add extra salt if desired.

**YIELD:** 1½ cups (375 mL)
**EXCHANGE:** 1 lean meat
1 milk
¼ bread
**CALORIES:** 220

# Kidney Stew

| | | |
|---|---|---|
| 2 ounces | beef kidney (cooked) | 60 g |
| 1½ cups | beef broth | 375 mL |
| 3 T. | leek (chopped) | 45 mL |
| 1 slice | bacon (cooked and drained) | 1 slice |
| ¼ cup | mushrooms | 60 mL |
| 3 T. | green pepper (sliced) | 45 mL |
| dash each | parsley, thyme, tarragon, salt, pepper | dash each |

Heat all ingredients to a boil. Reduce heat and simmer until green pepper slices are tender.

**YIELD:** 1½ cups (375 mL)  **CALORIES:** 130
**EXCHANGE:** 2 lean meat
1 fat

# Pizza Stew

| | | |
|---|---|---|
| 1 ounce | Canadian bacon | 30 g |
| 1 ½ cups | Tomato Sauce (p. 143) | 375 mL |
| ¼ cup | water 60 mL | |
| 2 tablespoons | onion (chopped) | 30 mL |
| 1 tablespoon | mushroom pieces | 15 mL |
| 1 tablespoon | black olives (pitted and chopped) | 15 mL |
| 1 tablespoon | celery (chopped) | 15 mL |
| 1 tablespoon | green pepper (chopped) | 15 mL |
| dash each | oregano, garlic powder, salt to taste | |
| ½ cup | elbow macaroni (cooked) | 125 mL |

Fry Canadian bacon; drain and cut away any fat. Heat Tomato Sauce and water to a boil. Add bacon, vegetables, and seasonings. Cook until vegetables are tender. Add macaroni; reheat.

**YIELD:** 2¼ cups (560 mL)
**EXCHANGE:** 1 high-fat meat
1 bread
1 vegetable
**CALORIES:** 275

# Bean Stew

| | | |
|---|---|---|
| 1 T. | pinto beans | 15 mL |
| 1 T. | northern beans | 15 mL |
| 1 T. | lentils | 15 mL |
| 1 cup | beef broth | 250 mL |
| 1 T. | carrot (sliced) | 15 mL |
| 1 T. | hominy | 15 mL |
| 1 t. | onion (diced) | 5 mL |
| ½ t. | green chilies (chopped) | 2 mL |
| dash each | garlic powder, oregano, salt, pepper | dash each |

Boil beans and lentils in beef broth for 10 minutes, covered. Allow to stand 1 to 2 hours, or overnight. Place softened beans and remaining ingredients in baking dish. Bake at 350° F (175° C) for 45 minutes to 1 hour, or until ingredients are tender.

Microwave:  Place beans and lentils in beef broth; cover. Cook on High for 5 minutes. Allow to stand 1 to 2 hours or overnight. Add remaining ingredients. Cook on Medium for 10 to 15 minutes, or until ingredients are tender.

**YIELD:**      1½ cups (375 mL)
**EXCHANGE:**  1 lean meat
             2 bread
**CALORIES:**   225

# Zucchini Meatball Stew

| | | |
|---|---|---|
| 1 ounce | ground beef | 30 g |
| ½ cup | ground zucchini | 125 mL |
| 1 teaspoon | onion (finely chopped) | 5 mL |
| 1 | egg | 1 |
| ¼ cup | rice (uncooked) | 60 mL |
| dash each | oregano, cumin, garlic salt, pepper | dash each |
| 1 cup | beef broth | 250 mL |
| 1 large | tomato (diced) | 1 large |
| 1 teaspoon | parsley (chopped) | 5 mL |
| | salt and pepper to taste | |

Combine ground beef, zucchini, onion, egg, rice, and seasonings; mix thoroughly. Shape into small meatballs. Combine beef broth, tomato, and parsley in saucepan; heat to boil. Drop meatballs into hot broth, one at a time. Cover and simmer 30 to 40 minutes. Add salt and pepper.

**MICROWAVE:**  Cook beef broth, tomato, and parsley on High for 3 minutes, covered. Drop meatballs into broth. Cook on High 5 minutes. Hold 10 minutes. Add salt and pepper.

**YIELD:**     1¾ cups (430 mL)
**EXCHANGE:** 2 medium-fat meat
              1 vegetable
              1 bread
**CALORIES:** 203

# Chicken Giblet Stew

| | | |
|---|---|---|
| 3 ounces | chicken giblets | 90 g |
| 2 cups | water | 500 mL |
| ¼ teaspoon | thyme | 2 mL |
| ¼ | bay leaf | ¼ |
| ⅛ teaspoon | parsley (crushed) | 1 mL |
| | salt and pepper to taste | |
| 3 tablespoons | potatoes (diced) | 45 mL |
| 2 tablespoons | onion (diced) | 30 mL |
| 2 tablespoons | celery (diced) | 30 mL |
| 2 tablespoons | green beans (sliced) | 30 mL |
| 2 tablespoons | carrots (diced) | 30 mL |
| 2 tablespoons | peas | 30 mL |
| 1 teaspoon | flour | 5 mL |
| ¼ cup | water | 60 mL |

Remove center muscle of giblets. Place the 2 cups water, giblets, and seasonings in saucepan; cover. Heat to a boil; reduce heat and simmer until giblets are tender, about 1 hour. Add extra water to make about 2 cups (500 mL) liquid. Remove bay leaf. Add vegetables; reheat and cook until vegetables are tender. Blend flour with the ¼ cup water. Blend into stew. Cook to desired thickness.

**YIELD:**                 3 servings, 1 cup (250 mL) each
**EXCHANGE 1 SERVING:**   1 lean meat
                          1 bread
                          1 vegetable
**CALORIES 1 SERVING:**   120

# Pepper Pot
### (Leftovers may be used)

| | | |
|---|---|---|
| 2 ounces | lean pork, cut in 1-inch (2.5-cm) cubes | 60 g |
| 1 ounce | beef, cut in 1-inch (2.5-cm) cubes | 30 g |
| 1 ounce | chicken, cut in 1-inch (2.5-cm) cubes | 30 g |
| ¼ cup | carrot pieces | 60 mL |
| ¼ cup | onion slices | 60 mL |
| ¼ cup | celery pieces | 60 mL |
| ¼ cup | potatoes (cubed) | 60 mL |
| ½ cup | water | 125 ml |
| 1 t. | flour | 5 mL |
| dash each | curry powder, garlic powder, salt, pepper | dash each |

Brown pork and beef cubes slowly in frying pan. Add chicken cubes for last few minutes; drain. Place meat, carrots, onions, celery, and potatoes in individual baking dish. Combine water, flour, and seasonings in screw top jar; shake to blend well. Pour over meat mixture. Cover tightly and bake at 350° F (175° C) for 45 minutes to 1 hour, or until meat is tender and gravy has thickened.

**MICROWAVE:** Reduce water to ¼ cup (60 mL). Cover. Cook on High for 10 minutes. Hold 5 minutes.

| | |
|---|---|
| YIELD: | 1 serving |
| EXCHANGE: | 4 high-fat meat |
| | 1 vegetable |
| | 1 bread |
| CALORIES: | 418 |

# Stefado

| | | |
|---|---|---|
| 1 stick | cinnamon | 1 stick |
| 1 | bay leaf | 1 |
| 5 whole | cloves | 5 |
| 12 ounces | beef roast (cubed) | 360 g |
| | Salt and pepper to taste | |
| 1 teaspoon | margarine | 5 mL |
| 1½ cups | onions (sliced) | 375 mL |
| 3 medium | tomatoes (peeled and cubed) | 3 medium |
| ½ cup | red wine | 125 mL |
| 1 teaspoon | brown sugar replacement | 5 mL |
| 2 tablespoons | raisins | 30 mL |
| 1 cup | water | 250 mL |
| 1 | garlic clove (crushed) | 1 |

Place cinnamon, bay leaf, and cloves in small cheesecloth bag. Combine with remaining ingredients in soup kettle; cook 1 to 1½ hours until meat is tender. Remove spice bag before serving.

**MICROWAVE:** Same as above. Cook on High 15 to 20 minutes.

| | |
|---|---|
| **YIELD:** | 3 servings, 1 cup (250 mL) each |
| **EXCHANGE 1 SERVING:** | 4 high-fat meat |
| | 1 vegetable |
| **CALORIES 1 SERVING:** | 430 |

# CASSEROLES AND ONE-DISH MEALS

## Beef Stroganoff

| | | |
|---|---|---|
| 3 ounces | lean beef (cubed) | 90 g |
| 1 teaspoon | margarine | 5 mL |
| ½ | onion (cut into large pieces) | ½ |
| ¼ teaspoon | garlic (minced) | 1 mL |
| 2 tablespoons | mushroom pieces | 30 mL |
| ½ cup | condensed cream of mushroom soup | 125 mL |
| 1 tablespoon | lo-cal sour cream | 15 mL |
| 1 teaspoon | ketchup | 5 mL |
| dash each | Worcestershire sauce, ground bay leaf, salt, pepper | dash each |
| 1 cup | noodles | 250 mL |

Brown beef cubes in margarine. Add onion, garlic, and mushrooms. Cook over low heat until onion is partially cooked; remove from heat. Combine condensed soup, sour cream, ketchup, and seasonings; blend well. Pour over beef mixture; heat thoroughly. Do not boil. Serve over noodles.

**YIELD:** 1 serving
**EXCHANGE:** 3 high-fat meat
2½ bread
**CALORIES:** 470

# Packaged Steak Supper

| | | |
|---|---|---|
| 3 ounces | beef minute steak | 90 g |
| 1 small | potato | 1 small |
| 2 tablespoons | carrot (sliced) | 30 mL |
| 2 tablespoons | onion (sliced) | 30 mL |
| 2 tablespoons | celery (sliced) | 30 mL |
| 2 large | tomato slices | 2 large |
| | salt and pepper to taste | |

Place steak on large piece of aluminum foil. Layer vegetables in order given. Add salt and pepper. Wrap in foil, sealing ends securely. Bake at 350° F (175° C) for 1 hour.

**MICROWAVE:** Place in plastic wrap. Cook on High for 10 minutes.

**YIELD:** 1 serving
**EXCHANGE:** 3 medium-fat meat
1 bread
½ vegetable
**CALORIES:** 375

# Quick Kabobs

| | | |
|---|---|---|
| 2 oz. | cooked roast beef, cut in 1-inch cubes | 60 g |
| 6 | 1-inch (2.5-cm) green pepper squares | 6 |
| 6 | cherry tomatoes | 6 |
| 6 | 1-inch (2.5-cm) zucchini cubes | 6 |
| 6 | unsweetened pineapple chunks | 6 |
| 2 T | lo-cal French dressing | 6 |

Alternate beef, vegetables, and fruit on 2 skewers. Brush with 1 tablespoon (15 mL) of the French dressing. Broil 5 to 6 inches (12 to 15 cm) from heat for 8 minutes. Brush with remaining French dressing. Broil 4 minutes longer.

**YIELD:** 1 serving (2 kabobs)
**EXCHANGE:** 2 medium-fat meat
1 vegetable
1 fruit
**CALORIES:** 150

# Beef and Rice Casserole

| | | |
|---|---|---|
| 3 ounces | ground beef | 90 g |
| 1 tablespoon | onion (chopped) | 15 mL |
| 1 tablespoon | celery (chopped) | 15 mL |
| ¾ cup | condensed chicken gumbo soup | 180 mL |
| ¼ cup | water | 60 mL |
| ½ cup | rice (uncooked) | 125 mL |
| ¼ cup | condensed cream of mushroom soup | 60 mL |
| | salt and pepper to taste | |

Combine ground beef, onion, and celery with a small amount of water in a saucepan. Boil until onion is tender; drain. Combine condensed chicken gumbo soup, water, and rice. Simmer until all moisture is absorbed. Mix beef mixture, rice, and mushroom soup; pour into a small greased casserole dish. Add salt and pepper. Bake at 350° F (175° C) for 25 minutes.

**MICROWAVE:** Cook on Medium for 8 to 10 minutes

**YIELD:** 1 serving
**EXCHANGE:** 3 high-fat meat
2 bread
**CALORIES:** 380

# German Goulash

| | | |
|---|---|---|
| 3 ounces | lean ground beef | 90 g |
| 1 teaspoon | onion (chopped) | 5 mL |
| 1 tablespoon | green pepper (chopped) | 15 mL |
| 1 tablespoon | celery (chopped) | 15 mL |
| ¼ | bay leaf (crushed) | ¼ |
| ½ cup | kidney beans (cooked) | 125 mL |
| ½ cup | elbow macaroni (cooked) | 125 mL |
| ¼ cup | carrot (sliced) | 60 mL |
| | salt and pepper to taste | |

Brown ground beef, onion, green pepper, and celery over low heat; drain. Add crushed bay leaf, kidney beans, macaroni, and carrots; mix gently. Add salt and pepper. Pour into casserole dish; cover. Bake at 350° F (175° C) for 40 minutes.

**MICROWAVE:** Cook on Medium for 7 minutes.

**YIELD:** 1 serving
**EXCHANGE:** 3 medium-fat meat
2 ½ bread
**CALORIES:** 413

# Stuffed Peppers

| | | |
|---|---|---|
| 1 | green pepper | 1 |
| 2 tablespoons | rice | 30 mL |
| 2 ounces | lean ground beef | 60 g |
| 1 | egg | 1 |
| 1 teaspoon | onion flakes | 5 mL |
| 1 tablespoon | mushrooms (finely chopped) | 15 mL |
| | salt and pepper to taste | |
| 1 teaspoon | Tomato Sauce (p. 128) | 5 mL |

Cut green pepper in half, lengthwise. Remove membrane and seeds; rinse, drain, and reserve shells. Boil rice with ½ cup (125 mL) of water for 5 minutes; drain. Combine ground beef, rice, egg, onion flakes, and mushrooms; blend thoroughly. Add salt and pepper. Fill green pepper cavities with beef mixture; top with Tomato Sauce. Place in baking dish; cover. Bake at 350° F (175° C) for 20 to 25 minutes.

**MICROWAVE:** Cook on High for 10 minutes.

| | |
|---|---|
| **YIELD:** | 1 serving |
| **EXCHANGE:** | 3 medium-fat meat |
| | 1 bread |
| | 1 vegetable |
| **CALORIES:** | 255 |

# Lasagne

| | | |
|---|---|---|
| 2 ounces | ground beef | 60 g |
| 1 tablespoon | onion (chopped) | 15 mL |
| ½ cup | Tomato Sauce (P. 128) | 125 mL |
| 3 tablespoons | water | 45 mL |
| ¼ teaspoon | garlic powder | 1 mL |
| ½ teaspoon | oregano | 3 mL |
| | salt and pepper to taste | |
| 1½ cups | lasagne noodles (cooked) | 375 mL |
| 1 ounce | mozzarella cheese (grated) | 30 g |
| 1 ounce | provolone cheese (grated) | 30 g |

Crumble beef in small amount of water; add onion. Boil until meat is cooked; drain. Blend Tomato Sauce, 3 tablespoons (45 mL) water, garlic powder, oregano, salt, and pepper. Add beef-onion mixture; stir to blend. Spread small amount of sauce into bottom of individual baking dish.

Layer noodles, sauce, mozzarella and provolone cheese. Bake at 375° F (190° C) for 30 minutes.

**MICROWAVE:**    Cook on High for 10 minutes.

| | |
|---|---|
| **YIELD:** | 1 serving |
| **EXCHANGE:** | 4 high-fat meat |
| | 3 bread |
| **CALORIES:** | 485 |

# Hamburger Pie

| | | |
|---|---|---|
| 2 pounds | lean ground beef | 1 kg |
| ½ cup | cornflakes (crushed) | 125 mL |
| ¼ teaspoon | garlic powder | 1 mL |
| ½ teaspoon | onion (finely chopped) | 3 mL |
| 1 | egg | 1 |
| | salt and pepper to taste | |
| 2¼ cups | water | 560 mL |
| 1 cup | skim milk | 250 mL |
| 1 teaspoon | salt | 5 mL |
| 2 cups | instant mashed potatoes | 500 mL |
| 1 teaspoon | margarine | 5 mL |

Combine ground beef, cornflakes, garlic powder, onion, and egg; mix well. Add salt and pepper. Place beef mixture in 9-inch (23-cm) pie pan. Pat to cover bottom and sides evenly. Bake at 425° F (220° C) for 30 minutes; drain off excess fat. Heat water, skim milk, and salt just to a boil; remove from heat. Add potato granules; mix thoroughly. Add margarine; blend well. Cover and allow to stand 5 minutes, or until potatoes thicken. Spread evenly over meat mixture. Return to oven and bake until potatoes are golden brown. Allow to rest 10 minutes before cutting pie into wedges.

**MICROWAVE:** Cover beef mixture. Cook on Medium for 10 to 12 minutes; drain. Cover with potatoes. Cook on Medium for 2 minutes. Hold 5 minutes.

**YIELD:** 8 servings
**EXCHANGE 1 SERVING:** 4 high-fat meat
1 bread
½ fat
**CALORIES 1 SERVING:** 372

# Wiener-Egg Scramble

| | | |
|---|---|---|
| 1 slice | bacon | 1 slice |
| 1 teaspoon | onion (chopped) | 5 mL |
| 1 | wiener (sliced) | 1 |
| ½ teaspoon | green pepper (chopped) | 2 mL |
| 1 | egg | 1 |
| 1 teaspoon | skim milk | 5 mL |
| dash | Worcestershire sauce | dash |

Cook bacon until crisp; drain bacon and pan. Crumble bacon. Place bacon, onion, wiener, and green pepper in pan. Saute on low heat until onion is tender. Beat egg with skim milk and Worcestershire sauce; pour over wiener mixture. Cook until set.

**YIELD:** 1 serving
**EXCHANGE:** 2 high-fat meat
2 fat
**CALORIES:** 170

# Cheese Lasagne

| | | |
|---|---|---|
| ½ cup | Tomato Sauce (p. 143) | 125 mL |
| 3 tablespoons | water | 45 mL |
| 1 tablespoon | onion | 15 mL |
| ¼ teaspoon | garlic powder | 1 mL |
| ½ teaspoon | oregano | 3 mL |
| | salt and pepper to taste | |
| ¼ cup | large curd cottage cheese | 60 mL |
| 1 | egg | 1 |
| 1½ cups | lasagne noodles (cooked) | 375 mL |
| 2 ounces | mozzarella cheese | 60 g |
| 1 tablespoon | parmesan cheese | 15 mL |

Combine Tomato Sauce, water, onion, garlic powder, oregano, salt, and pepper. Thoroughly blend together cottage cheese and egg. Spread small amount of sauce into bottom of individual baking dish. Alternate layers of noodles, sauce, cottage cheese mixture, and mozzarella cheese. Top with Parmesan cheese. Bake at 375° F (190° C) for 30 minutes.

**MICROWAVE:** Cook on High for 10 minutes.

**YIELD:** 1 serving
**EXCHANGE:** 3 high-fat meat
3 bread
**CALORIES:** 350

# Clam Pilaf

| | | |
|---|---|---|
| 2 ounces | clams (minced) | 60 g |
| ½ cup | rice (cooked) | 125 mL |
| 2 T. | onion (chopped) | 30 mL |
| 1 medium | fresh tomato (peeled and cubed) | 1 medium |
| dash | each ground bay leaf, thyme, salt, pepper | dash |
| 2 T. | grated Cheddar cheese | 30 mL |

Combine clams, rice, onion, tomato, and seasonings in baking dish; top with cheese. Bake at 350° F (175° C) for 25 minutes.

**MICROWAVE:** Combine clams, rice, onion, tomato, and seasonings. Cook on High for 5 minutes; top with cheese. Reheat on High for 1 minute.

**YIELD:** 1 serving
**EXCHANGE:** 2 lean meat
1 bread
**CALORIES:** 170

# Macaroni and Cheese Supreme

| | | |
|---|---|---|
| 1 cup | elbow macaroni | 250 mL |
| 11-oz. can | condensed cream of mushroom soup | 300-g can |
| 6 ounces | cheese (shredded) | 180 mL |
| 1 teaspoon | yellow mustard | 5 mL |
| 1 teaspoon | salt | 5 mL |
| dash | pepper | dash |
| 2 cups | cooked spinach (drained) | 500 mL |
| 12 ounces | lean meat (diced) | 360 g |

Cook macaroni as directed on package; drain. Combine mushroom soup, cheese, mustard, salt, and pepper. Add macaroni; stir well. Spread cooked spinach on bottom of lightly greased 13 x 9-inch (33 x 23-cm) baking dish. Top with meat. Spoon macaroni mixture evenly over entire surface. Bake at 375° F (190° C) for 40 minutes. Allow to cool 15 minutes before serving.

**MICROWAVE:** Cook on Medium for 12 to 15 minutes. Turn dish halfway through cooking time. Allow to rest 15 minutes before serving.

# Turkey à la King I

| | | |
|---|---|---|
| 1 tablespoon | green pepper (diced) | 15 mL |
| 2 tablespoons | celery (sliced) | 30 mL |
| ¼ cup | condensed cream of chicken soup | 60 mL |
| 2 tablespoons | skim milk | 30 mL |
| 2 tablespoons | mushrooms (chopped) | 30 mL |
| 3 ounces | cooked turkey (diced) | 90 g |
| 1 tablespoon | pimiento (chopped) | 15 mL |
| | salt and pepper to taste | |
| 2 slices | bread (toasted) | 2 slices |

Cook green pepper and celery in boiling water until tender; drain. Blend condensed soup and skim milk. Add green pepper, celery, mushrooms, turkey, and pimiento. Add salt and pepper. Heat slightly over low heat. Cut toast into triangles; place in small bowl, tips up. Spoon turkey mixture over tips.

**YIELD:**     1 serving
**EXCHANGE:**  3 medium-fat meat
               2 ¼ bread
               ¼ vegetable
**CALORIES:**  450

# Turkey à la King II

| | | |
|---|---|---|
| ¼ cup | White Sauce (p. 149) | 60 mL |
| 1 ounce | cooked turkey (diced) | 30 g |
| ¼ cup | mushroom pieces | 60 mL |
| 2 tablespoons | green pepper (chopped) | 30 mL |
| 1 tablespoon | stuffed green olives (chopped) | 15 mL |
| | salt and pepper to taste | |
| | dough for 1 baking powder biscuit (p. 97) | |

Heat White Sauce. Combine sauce, turkey, mushrooms, green pepper, and olives; add salt and pepper. Pour into lightly greased individual baking dish. Top with biscuit dough. Bake at 375° F (190° C) for 15 to 20 minutes, or until biscuit is golden brown.

**YIELD:** 1 serving
**EXCHANGE:** 1 medium-fat meat
1 vegetable
1 bread
**CALORIES:** 168

# Chicken Gambeano

| | | |
|---|---|---|
| ¼ cup | condensed cream of chicken soup | 60 mL |
| 3 tablespoons | skim milk | 45 mL |
| ¼ cup | zucchini (cubed) | 60 mL |
| ¼ cup | green beans | 60 mL |
| 2 ounces | cooked chicken (cubed) | 60 g |
| ¼ teaspoon | poultry seasoning | 2 mL |
| | salt and pepper to taste | |
| 1¼ cups | linguine (cooked) | 310 mL |

Blend condensed soup and skim milk; place in saucepan. Add zucchini and green beans. Cook over medium heat until vegetables are partially tender. Add chicken and seasonings; reheat. Serve over linguine.

Microwave: Blend condensed soup and skim milk in bowl. Add zucchini and green beans; cover. Cook on High for 5 to 7 minutes, or until vegetables are partially tender. Add chicken and seasonings; reheat on Medium for 4 minutes. Serve over linguine.

**YIELD:** 1 serving
**EXCHANGE:** 3 bread
2 medium-fat meat
½ vegetable
**CALORIES:** 300

# Mostaccioli with Oysters

| | | |
|---|---|---|
| 8-ounce can | oysters with liquid (minced) | 225 g |
| 4-ounce can | mushroom pieces | 120 g |
| ½ cup | green pepper (sliced) | 125 mL |
| 1 tablespoon | parsley | 15 mL |
| 1 teaspoon | garlic powder | 5 mL |
| | salt and pepper to taste | |
| 3 cups | mostaccioli noodles (cooked) | 750 mL |

Combine minced oysters with liquid, mushrooms, green pepper, and parsley in saucepan. Add garlic powder. Cook until green pepper is crispy tender. Add salt and pepper. Serve over mostaccioli noodles.

**MICROWAVE:** Combine minced oysters with liquid, mushrooms, green pepper, parsley, and garlic powder in bowl. Cook on High for 4 minutes or until green pepper is crispy tender. Add salt and pepper. Serve over mostaccioli noodles.

**YIELD:** 2 servings
**EXCHANGE 1 SERVING:** 4 lean meat
1½ bread
**CALORIES 1 SERVING:** 195

# Fish Noodle Special

| | | |
|---|---|---|
| ¼ cup | condensed cream of celery soup | 60 mL |
| 2 T. | water | 30 mL |
| 2 T. | mushroom pieces | 30 mL |
| 2 T. | onion (finely chopped) | 30 mL |
| dash each | thyme, ground rosemary, salt, pepper | dash each |
| 1 cup | noodles (cooked) | 250 mL |
| 2 T. | peas | 30 mL |
| 3 ounces | cooked perch (flaked) | 90 g |

Blend condensed soup with water. Add mushrooms, onion, and seasonings; mix thoroughly. Combine noodles, peas, and perch in small baking dish. Pour soup mixture over entire surface; toss to mix. Bake at 350° F (175° C) for 30 minutes.

**MICROWAVE:** Cook on High for 5 to 6 minutes.

**YIELD:** 1 serving
**EXCHANGE:** 3 lean meat
2½ bread
**CALORIES:** 285

# Veal Steak Parmesan

| | | |
|---|---|---|
| 1 T. | flour | 15 mL |
| 1 t. | salt | 5 mL |
| dash each | poultry seasoning, salt, pepper, paprika | dash each |
| 4 ounces | veal steak (cut in half) | 120 g |
| 1 t. | shortening | 5 mL |
| ½ cup | wide noodles (cooked) | 125 mL |
| ½ cup | sour sream sauce, prepared | 125 mL |
| 3 T. | hot water | 45 mL |
| 1 t. | Parmesan cheese | 5 mL |

Combine flour, salt, and seasonings in shaker bag. Add veal steak; shake to coat. Remove veal from bag and shake off excess flour. Heat shortening in small skillet. Brown veal on both sides; place in small baking dish. Cover with noodles. Blend sour cream sauce and hot water. Pour over noodles. Top with Parmesan cheese. Bake at 350° F (175° C) for 45 minutes, or until veal is tender.

**MICROWAVE:** Cover. Cook on Medium to High for 15 minutes, or until meat is tender.

| | |
|---|---|
| **YIELD:** | 1 serving |
| **EXCHANGE:** | 4¼ medium-fat meat |
| | 2 bread |
| **CALORIES:** | 390 |

# Kole 'n Klump

| ½ cup | Brussels sprouts | 125 mL |
|---|---|---|
| 2 ounces | lean pork cubes | 60 g |
| pinch | caraway seeds, salt, pepper | pinch |
| ¼ cup | potato (grated) | 60 mL |
| ¼ teaspoon | onion salt | 1 mL |
| dash each | thyme, salt, pepper | dash each |

Boil Brussels sprouts, pork, caraway seeds, salt, and pepper with a small amount of water until partially cooked; drain. Place in individual baking dish. Cover with potato; sprinkle with onion salt, thyme, salt, and pepper. Cover tightly. Bake at 375° F (190° C) for 1 hour.

**MICROWAVE:** Cook on High for 10 to 12 minutes. Turn dish a quarter turn after 6 minutes.

YIELD:       1 serving
EXCHANGE:  1 bread
             2 high-fat meat
CALORIES:   232

# Ham and Scalloped Potatoes

| | | |
|---|---|---|
| 2 ounces | lean ham (diced) | 60 g |
| 1 medium | potato (peeled and sliced) | 1 medium |
| 2 tablespoons | onion | 30 mL |
| 2 teaspoons | parsley | 10 mL |
| | vegetable cooking spray | |
| ¼ cup | condensed cream of celery soup | 60 mL |
| ¼ cup | milk | 60 mL |
| | salt and pepper to taste | |

Combine ham, potato, onion, and parsley in baking dish coated with vegetable coking spray. Blend condensed soup and milk; pour over potato mixture; cover. Bake at 350° F (175° C) for 1 hour, or until potatoes are tender. Add salt and pepper.

**MICROWAVE:** Cook on high for 10 minutes, or until potatoes are tender. Add salt and pepper.

YIELD:       1 serving
EXCHANGE:  2 high-fat meat
             1½ bread
             ½ milk
CALORIES:   365

# Tuna Soufflé

| | | |
|---|---|---|
| 11-ounce can | condensed cream of celery soup | 300-g can |
| 2 teaspoons | parsley (finely chopped) | 10 mL |
| 1 teaspoon | salt | 5 mL |
| dash | pepper | dash |
| ½ teaspoon | marjoram | 3 mL |
| 7-ounce can | tuna (in water) | 200-g can |
| 6 | eggs (separated) | 6 |
| 1 cup | mixed vegetables (cooked) | 250 mL |

Combine condensed soup, parsley, salt, pepper, marjoram, and tuna in saucepan. Heat, stirring constantly, until mixture is hot. Remove from heat and cool slightly. Add egg yolks, one at a time, beating well after each addition. Stir in vegetables. Beat egg whites until soft peaks form. Fold small amount of beaten egg whites into egg yolk mixture then fold egg yolk mixture into remaining egg whites. Pour into lightly greased 10-inch (25-cm) soufflé dish. Bake at 325° F (165° C) for 50 minutes, or until firm and golden brown. Serve immediately.

| | |
|---|---|
| **YIELD:** | 8 servings |
| **EXCHANGE 1 SERVING:** | 1½ lean meat |
| | 1 bread |
| **CALORIES 1 SERVING:** | 134 |

# Hot Tuna Dish

| | | |
|---|---|---|
| ½ cup | condensed cream of chicken soup | 125 mL |
| 2 ounces | chunk tuna (in water) | 60 g |
| 2 tablespoons | celery (diced) | 30 mL |
| 1 tablespoon | onion (chopped) | 15 mL |
| 1 | egg (hard cooked) | 1 |
| 4 tablespoons | potato chips (crushed) | 60 mL |

Combine condensed soup, tuna, celery, and onion; mix thoroughly. Pour into small casserole. Slice egg; layer egg, then crushed potato chips. Bake at 350° F (175° C) for 20 minutes.

**MICROWAVE:** Cook on Medium for 7 to 10 minutes.

| | |
|---|---|
| **YIELD:** | 1 serving |
| **EXCHANGE:** | 1⅓ bread |
| | 3 medium-fat meat |
| **CALORIES:** | 297 |

# Casserole of Shrimp

| | | |
|---|---|---|
| 2 teaspoons | margarine | 30 mL |
| 1 tablespoon | parsley (chopped) | 15 mL |
| 1 tablespoon | sherry | 15 mL |
| dash each | garlic powder, paprika, cayenne | dash each |
| ½ cup | soft bread crumbs | 125 mL |
| 3 ounces | large shrimp (cooked) | 90 g |

Melt margarine over low heat. Add parsley, sherry, and seasonings; cook slightly. Add bread crumbs; toss to mix. Place shrimp in small baking dish. Top with bread crumb mixture. Bake at 325° F (165° C) for 20 minutes.

**MICROWAVE:** Melt margarine; add parsley, sherry, and seasonings. Cook on High for 2 minutes. Add bread crumbs; toss to mix. Place shrimp in small baking dish. Top with bread crumb mixture. Cook on Medium for 5 to 7 minutes.

| | |
|---|---|
| **YIELD:** | 1 serving |
| **EXCHANGE:** | 3 high-fat meat |
| | 1 bread |
| **CALORIES:** | 204 |

# Stuffed Cabbage Rolls

| | | |
|---|---|---|
| 2 large | cabbage leaves | 2 large |
| 2 ounces | ground veal | 60 g |
| 2 ounces | lean ground beef | 60 g |
| 3 tablespoons | skim milk | 45 mL |
| 1 slice | dry bread (crumbled) | 1 slice |
| 1 teaspoon | onion (grated) | 5 mL |
| dash each | salt, pepper, nutmeg | dash each |
| ½ cup | beef broth | 125 mL |
| 1 tablespoon | flour | 15 mL |

Cook cabbage leaves in boiling salted water until tender; drain. Combine ground veal, beef, skim milk, bread crumbs, onion, salt, pepper, and nutmeg; mix thoroughly. Place half of meat mixture in a cabbage leaf and rollup, tucking ends in. Secure with toothpicks. Place in small baking dish. Repeat with remaining meat mixture and cabbage leaf. Blend beef broth and flour; pour over cabbage rolls. Bake at 350° F (175° C) for 45 to 50 minutes.

**MICROWAVE:** Cook on Medium for 10 to 12 minutes.

**YIELD:** 1 serving
**EXCHANGE:** 4 medium-fat meat
1 vegetable
1 bread
**CALORIES:** 396

# Hungarian Goulash

| | | |
|---|---|---|
| 1 tablespoon | shortening or margarine | 30 mL |
| 1 ounce | lean beef (diced) | 30 g |
| 1 ounce | lean veal (diced) | 30 g |
| 1 ounce | beef kidney (diced) | 30 g |
| 2 teaspoons | onion (chopped) | 10 mL |
| 1 teaspoon | green pepper (chopped) | 5 mL |
| 3 | cherry tomatoes (halved) | 3 |
| ½ cup | potato (diced) | 125 mL |
| ¼ cup | carrot (diced) | 60 mL |
| ¼ teaspoon | salt | 1 mL |
| dash each | paprika, pepper, marjoram | dash each |

Heat shortening or margarine in skillet; add meat. Brown on all sides; drain. Place in individual casserole. Add remaining ingredients. Add enough water to cover. Cover casserole tightly; bake at 350° F (175° C) for 1 hour.

**MICROWAVE:** Cook on high for 20 to 25 minutes. Stir halfway through cooking time.

**YIELD:** 1 serving
**EXCHANGE:** 3 high-fat meat
1 bread
1 vegetable
**CALORIES:** 348

# MEATS AND POULTRY

## Steak Roberto

| | | |
|---|---|---|
| ¼ cup | margarine | 60 mL |
| 1 teaspoon | garlic power | 5 mL |
| 1 pound | beef tenderloin (8 slices) | 500 g |
| ½ teaspoon | steak sauce | 3 mL |
| ¼ teaspoon | bay leaf (crushed) | 1 mL |
| 1 tablespoon | lemon juice | 15 mL |
| ½ teaspoon | salt | 2 mL |
| dash | pepper | dash |

Melt margarine and combine with garlic powder. Set aside for 20 minutes to allow flavor to develop. Heat 1 tablespoon (15 mL) of the garlic margarine in heavy skillet until very hot. Place as many beef tenderloin slices as possible in skillet; brown on both sides. Remove to warm steak platter. Repeat with remaining beef, if necessary. Reduce heat. Add remaining garlic margarine to pan. Add steak sauce, bay leaf, lemon juice, salt, and pepper; blend thoroughly. Pour over beef tenderloin on platter.

**YIELD:** 8 servings
**EXCHANGE 1 SERVING:** 2 medium-fat meat
½ fat
**CALORIES 1 SERVING:** 155

# Brisket of Beef with Horseradish

| | | |
|---|---|---|
| 3- to 4-pound | beef brisket | 1½- to 2-kg |
| | salt and pepper to taste | |
| 1 medium | onion (sliced) | 1 medium |
| 1 | bay leaf | 1 |
| 1 tablespoon | lemon juice | 15 mL |
| ½ cup | horseradish (grated) | 125 mL |
| | salt and pepper to taste | |

Place brisket in large kettle; add salt and pepper. Add onion, bay leaf, and enough water to cover brisket. Bring to a boil. Reduce heat and simmer for 2 hours. Remove brisket from water. Combine lemon juice and horseradish. Rub surface of brisket with horseradish mixture. Return brisket to kettle, cover. Cook 1 hour longer.

**EXCHANGE 1 OUNCE (30 G):**    1 medium-fat meat
**CALORIES 1 OUNCE (30 G):**    84

# Beef Fondue

| | | |
|---|---|---|
| 1 small | tomato | 1 small |
| 2 cups | beef broth | 500 mL |
| 1 | bay leaf | 1 |
| ½ teaspoon | rosemary (ground) | 2 mL |
| | sirloin steak (cut into bite-size cubes) | |

Peel and crush tomato. Place beef broth, tomato, bay leaf, and rosemary in saucepan; heat to a broil. Pour into fondue pot, keep hot with a burner. Place steak cubes on spear. Cook in hot broth to desired doneness.

**EXCHANGE 1 OUNCE (30 G):**    1 high-fat meat
**CALORIES 1 OUNCE (30 G):**    88
*Note:* Amount of steak used depends on number of servings required.

# Sauerbraten

| | | |
|---|---|---|
| 4 ounces | lean beef roast | 120 g |
| ½ cup | beef broth | 125 mL |
| ¼ cup | water | 60 mL |
| ¼ cup | cider vinegar | 60 mL |
| ¼ teaspoon | salt | 1 mL |
| dash | garlic powder | dash |
| 1 teaspoon | margarine | 5 mL |

Place beef in glass pan or bowl. Combine remaining ingredients, except margarine; pour over beef. Marinate 4 to 5 days in refrigerator. Turn beef at least once a day. Melt margarine in small skillet; add beef and brown. Reduce heat. Add half of the marinade to the skillet. Simmer until beef is tender.

**YIELD:** 1 serving
**EXCHANGE:** 4 medium-fat meat
**CALORIES:** 300

# Mushroom-Stuffed Pork Chops

| | | |
|---|---|---|
| 2 tablespoons | mushroom pieces | 30 mL |
| 1 teaspoon | onion (chopped) | 5 mL |
| ½ teaspoon | parsley (chopped) | 2 mL |
| 1 teaspoon | raisins (soaked) | 5 mL |
| ¼ teaspoon | nutmeg | 1 mL |
| 1 | double pork chop | 1 |

Combine ingredients for stuffing; stir to blend. Split meaty part of chop down to bone; do not split through bone. Fill with stuffing; secure with poultry pins. Place on baking sheet. Bake uncovered at 350° F (175° C) for 35 to 40 minutes, or until tender. Turn once.

YIELD: 1 chop
EXCHANGE 1 OUNCE (30 G): 1 high-fat meat
CALORIES 1 OUNCE (30 G): 109

# Teriyaki Pork Steak

|  | pork steak (thinly sliced) |  |
|---|---|---|
| ½ cup | soy sauce | 125 mL |
| 1 tablespoon | wine vinegar | 15 mL |
| 2 tablespoons | lemon juice | 30 mL |
| ¼ cup | water | 60 mL |
| 2 tablespoons | sugar replacement | 30 mL |
| 1 ½ teaspoons | ginger | 7 mL |
| ½ teaspoon | garlic powder | 2 mL |

Place slices of pork steak in shallow dish. Combine remaining ingredients; pour over pork. Marinate 1 to 2 hours; turn once. Broil pork 5 to 6 inches (12 to 15 cm) from heat, for 2-3 minutes per side. Turn and broil second side.

EXCHANGE 1 OUNCE (30 G): 1 medium-fat meat
CALORIES 1 OUNCE (30 G): 89

*Note:* Amount of steak used depends on number of servings required.

# Calf's Liver

| | | |
|---|---|---|
| 1 tablespoon | flour | 15 mL |
| ½ teaspoon | bay leaf (finely crushed) | 2 mL |
| ¼ teaspoon | nutmeg | 1 mL |
| | salt and pepper to taste | |
| ½ cup | beef broth | 125 mL |
| 3 ounces | calf's liver | 90 g |
| | vegetable cooking spray | |

Combine flour, bay leaf, nutmeg, salt, and pepper in shaker bag. Add liver; shake to coat. Remove liver from bag and shake off excess flour. Brown liver in heavy skillet coated with vegetable cooking spray. Reduce heat. Add beef broth; cover. Simmer for 25 to 30 minutes, or until tender.

**YIELD:** 1 serving
**EXCHANGE:** 3 lean meat
**CALORIES:** 132

# Calf's Brains

| | | |
|---|---|---|
| 1 | calf's brain (trimmed) | 1 |
| 2 tablespoons | lemon juice | 30 mL |
| 1 tablespoon | cider vinegar | 15 mL |
| 1 teaspoon | thyme | 5 mL |
| 1 | bay leaf | 1 |
| 1/3 cup | onion (chopped) | 90 mL |
| 1 | parsley sprig (chopped) | 1 |
| 1/3 cup | celery (chopped) | 90 mL |

Rinse brain thoroughly. Cover with water. Add lemon juice and marinate for 2 to 4 hours. Drain. Cover with cold water. Add remaining ingredients. Bring to boil. Cover and simmer for 20 to 25 minutes, or until thoroughly cooked.

Remove from heat. Allow to rest 15 minutes. Remove brain from water. Slice thin.

**YIELD:** 1 brain
**EXCHANGE 1 OUNCE (30 G):** 1 lean meat
**CALORIES 1 OUNCE (30 G):** 45

# Veal Roast

| | | |
|---|---|---|
| 2- to 3-pound | veal roast | 1- to 1½-kg |
| 2 cups | beef broth | 500 mL |
| 1 medium | onion (sliced) | 1 medium |
| 1 | bay leaf | 1 |
| ¼ teaspoon | thyme | 1 mL |
| | salt and pepper to taste | |

Place roast in heavy kettle or roasting pan. Combine remaining ingredients. Pour over roast. Bake at 375° F (190° C) for 2 to 2½ hours, or until meat is very tender. While baking, baste with pan juices.

**EXCHANGE 1 OUNCE (30 G):** 1 lean meat
**CALORIES 1 OUNCE (30 G):** 55

# Veal Scaloppine

| | | |
|---|---|---|
| 2 ounces | veal steak (boned) | 60 g |
| ¼ cup | tomato (sieved) | 60 mL |
| 2 tablespoons | green pepper (chopped) | 30 mL |
| 1 tablespoon | mushroom pieces | 15 mL |
| 1 tablespoon | onions (chopped) | 15 mL |
| ¼ teaspoon | parsley | 1 mL |
| dash each | garlic powder, oregano | dash each |
| | salt and pepper to taste | |

Place veal on bottom of individual baking dish. Add remaining ingredients; cover.  bake at 350° F (175° C) for 45 minutes, or until meat is tender.

**MICROWAVE:** Cook on High for 10 to 12 minutes.  Turn and uncover last 2 minutes.

**YIELD:**      1 serving
**EXCHANGE:**  2 lean meat
                1 vegetable
**CALORIES:**   164

# Veal Scaloppine II

| ½ teaspoon | margarine | 3 mL |
| 2 ounces | veal round steak (thinly sliced) | 60 g |
| 2 tablespoons | tomato paste | 30 mL |
| 6 tablespoons | water | 90 mL |
| dash each | salt, pepper, oregano, garlic powder | |
| 1 tablespoon | mushrooms (sliced) | 15 mL |
| 1 teaspoon | onion (chopped) | 5 mL |
| 1 cup | spaghetti (cooked) | 250 mL |

Melt margarine in small skillet. Brown both sides of slices of veal steak. Place in small baking dish. Blend tomato paste, water, seasonings, mushrooms, and onion together. Pour over veal; cover. Bake at 350° F (175° C) for 30 minutes. Place veal on top of spaghetti. Pour sauce over all.

**MICROWAVE:** Cook covered on Medium for 12 minutes.

**YIELD:** 1 serving
**EXCHANGE:** 2 medium-fat meat
                2 bread
**CALORIES:** 310

# Veal Roll

| | | |
|---|---|---|
| 1 ounce | veal (thin slice) | 30 g |
| | salt and pepper to taste | |
| ½ ounce | prosciutto (thin slice) | 15 g |
| ½ ounce | Swiss cheese (thin slice) | 15 g |
| | vegetable cooking spray | |

Pound veal slice with mallet or edge of plate until very thin. Add salt and pepper. Place proscuitto on top and roll up. Secure with poultry pin. Brown in heavy skillet coated with vegetable cooking spray. Top with cheese slice. Cover. Cook over low heat just until cheese melts slightly. Serve on hot plate.

**YIELD:** 1 serving
**EXCHANGE:** 2 medium-fat meat
**CALORIES:** 156

# Beef Tongue

| | | |
|---|---|---|
| 1 | beef tongue | 1 |

Place tongue in large kettle; cover with water. Add 1 teaspoon (5 mL) salt per quart (L) of water. Bring to boil; reduce heat and simmer 3½ to 4 hours. Remove tongue; immediately place in ice water. Allow to soak 5 minutes. Remove skin and trim. Slice thin. Use for sandwiches.

**EXCHANGE 1 OUNCE (30 G):** 1 lean mat
**CALORIES 1 OUNCE (30 G):** 51

# Meat Loaf

| | | |
|---|---|---|
| 2 pounds | lean ground beef | 1 kg |
| ¼ cup | onion (grated) | 60 mL |
| 1 cup | soft bread crumbs | 250 mL |
| 1 | egg | 1 |
| ¼ cup | parsley (finely snipped) | 60 mL |
| 1¼ | teaspoons salt 6 mL | |
| dash | each pepper, thyme, marjoram | dash each |
| 1 teaspoon | evaporated milk | 5 mL |

Combine all ingredients. Add just enough water to form firm ball. Press into baking dish. Bake at 350° F (175° C) for 1½ hours.

**MICROWAVE:** Cook on High for 15 minutes. Turn dish halfway through cooking time. Allow to rest for 5 minutes before serving.

| | |
|---|---|
| **YIELD:** | 12 servings |
| **EXCHANGE 1 SERVING:** | 2½ high-fat meat |
| | ¼ bread |
| **CALORIES 1 SERVING:** | 237 |

# Klip Klops

| | | |
|---|---|---|
| 4 slices | bread (crust removed) | 4 slices |
| ½ cup | skim milk | 125 mL |
| ½ teaspoon | garlic powder | 2 mL |
| 1 teaspoon | onion salt | 5 mL |
| 1 pound | lean ground beef | 500 g |
| 1 | egg (beaten) | 1 |
| 1 quart | water | 1 L |
| 1 small | bay leaf | 1 small |
| 1 teaspoon | salt | 5 mL |
| 1 | clove | 1 |

Soak bread in skim milk. Add garlic powder, onion salt, ground beef, and egg; mix thoroughly. Form into 8 balls. Combine water, bay leaf, salt, and clove. Bring to boil. Drop balls into boiling water. Cook until beef is done (about 15 minutes). Drain before placing on hot platter.

**YIELD:**                8 servings
**EXCHANGE 1 SERVING:**   2 high-fat meat
                                 1 bread
**CALORIES 1 SERVING:**   190

# Roast Leg of Lamb

| | | |
|---|---|---|
| 5- to 6-pound | leg of lamb | 2½- to 3-kg |
| ½ cup | lo-cal Italian dressing | 125 mL |
| ½ cup | water | 125 mL |
| 3 tablespoons | lemon juice | 45 mL |
| 1 teaspoon | garlic powder | 5 mL |
| ½ teaspoon | rosemary (ground) | 2 mL |
| ½ teaspoon | thyme | 2 mL |
| ½ teaspoon | mace | 2 mL |
| 1 teaspoon | salt | 5 mL |
| ¼ teaspoon | pepper | 1 mL |

Wipe lamb with damp cloth. Puncture lamb with long, sharp spear or poultry pin. Place on a rack in roasting pan, fat side up. Blend remaining ingredients; pour over lamb. Roast uncovered at 325° F (165° C) for 3 to 3½ hours. Baste with pan juices every ½ hour. Add more Italian dressing and water, if necessary.

**EXCHANGE 1 OUNCE (30 G):**   1 medium-fat meat
**CALORIES 1 OUNCE (30 G):**   75

# Steak Hawaiian

| | | |
|---|---|---|
| 3 ounces | beef top round steak (sliced) | 90 g |
| ½ teaspoon | mace | 2 mL |
| 2 tablespoons | unsweetened pineapple juice | 30 mL |
| 1 | pineapple slice (unsweetened) | 1 |

Pound slices of round steak with mallet or edge of plate until thin. Sprinkle both sides with mace. Place in aluminum foil. Sprinkle with pineapple juice; top with pineapple slice. Secure foil tightly. Place in baking dish. Bake at 350° F (175° C) for 40 to 45 minutes.

**MICROWAVE:** Place in plastic wrap. Cook on High for 10 to 12 minutes.

**YIELD:** 1 serving
**EXCHANGE:** 3 lean meat
1 fruit
**CALORIES:** 200

# Lamb Shish Kebab

| | | |
|---|---|---|
| 4 pounds | lean lamb | 2 kg |
| 3 | garlic cloves (crushed) | 3 |
| 1½ teaspoons | salt | 7 mL |
| 1 | bay leaf | 1 |
| ½ teaspoon | pepper | 3 mL |
| ½ teaspoon | ground allspice | 3 mL |
| ½ teaspoon | ground clove | 3 mL |
| 1 teaspoon | white vinegar | 5 mL |
| 1 cup | skim milk | 250 mL |

Cut lamb into 2-inch (5-cm) cubes. Combine remaining ingredients; blend thoroughly. Pour over lamb in large bowl;

cover. Refrigerate overnight. Place lamb pieces on skewers. Barbecue or broil 10 to 15 minutes. Turn once.

**EXCHANGE 1 OUNCE (30 G):**   1 medium-fat meat
**CALORIES 1 OUNCE (3 G):**   89

# Swiss Steak

| | | |
|---|---|---|
| 1 teaspoon | margarine | 5 mL |
| 3 ounces | beef minute steak | 90 g |
| | salt and pepper to taste | |
| ¼ cup | celery (sliced) | 60 mL |
| 1 tablespoon | onion (chopped) | 15 mL |
| ¼ cup | tomato (crushed) | 60 mL |
| ¼ cup | water | 60 mL |

Heat margarine until very hot. Salt and pepper the steak. Brown both sides; drain. Place in individual baking dish. Add salt, pepper, and remaining ingredients. Cover. Bake at 375° F (175° C) for 1 hour, or until steak is tender.

**MICROWAVE:** Cook on High 8 to 10 minutes. Uncover last minute.

**YIELD:**   1 serving
**EXCHANGE:**   3 medium-fat meat
        1 fat
**CALORIES:**   220

# Roast Duck with Orange Sauce

| 4- to 5-pound | duck | 2- to 3- kg |
| 2 medium | oranges | 2 medium |
| | salt to taste | |
| | Orange Sauce (p. 149–150) | |

Wash inside and outside of duck thoroughly. Remove any fat from tail or neck opening. Salt interior of bird. Cut each orange (with peel) into 8 sections. Place inside the duck. Secure tail and neck skin, legs and wings with poultry pins. Salt exterior of duck. Place breast side up on a rack in roasting pan. Bake at 350° F (175° C) for 4 hours. During the final hour, baste with Orange Sauce every 15 minutes.

**EXCHANGE 1 OUNCE (30 G):**   1 high-fat meat
**CALORIES 1 OUNCE (30 G):**   96

# Roast Goose

| 5- to 6-pound | goose | 2½- to 3-kg |
| | salt to taste | |

Wash and dry goose thoroughly. Salt cavity and exterior. Fill cavity loosely with stuffing. Close cavity and secure tightly. Place breast side up in roasting pan. Roast at 350° F (175° C) for 30 to 40 minutes per pound, or about 3 to 4 hours. Cover with a loose tent of aluminum foil for the last hour to prevent excessive browning.

**YIELD:**   8 to 10 servings
**EXCHANGE 1 OUNCE (30 G):**   1 high-fat meat (without skin)
**CALORIES 1 OUNCE (30 G):**   20 (without skin)

*Note:* Add exchanges and calories for stuffing.

# Pollo Lesso

| | | |
|---|---|---|
| 3 ounces | chicken breast (boned) | 90 g |
| ½ | tomato (cut in 4 pieces) | ½ |
| ¼ | cucumber (peeled and sliced) | ¼ |
| ¼ cup | peas | 60 mL |
| dash each | salt, pepper, parsley | dash each |

Remove skin from chicken breast; boil chicken in small amount of salted water until almost tender. Add tomato pieces, cucumber slices, and peas. Heat thoroughly; drain. Place on serving plate. Sprinkle with salt, pepper, and parsley.

**MICROWAVE:** Place skinned chicken beast in individual dish; cover with plastic wrap. Cook on High for 12 minutes. Drain off any moisture. Add vegetables. Sprinkle with salt, pepper, and parsley. Cook on Medium for 4 minutes.

**YIELD:** 1 serving
**EXCHANGE:** 3 lean meat
1 bread
**CALORIES:** 202

# Giblet-Stuffed Chicken

| | | |
|---|---|---|
| 2 | giblets | 2 |
| 1 teaspoon | margarine | 5 mL |
| 2 tablespoons | rice | 30 mL |
| 1 tablespoon | raisins | 15 mL |
| 1 tablespoon | unsalted peanuts | 15 mL |
| | salt and pepper to taste | |
| 3 ounces | chicken breast (skinned and boned) | 90 g |

Simmer giblets in boiling water for 1 hour, or until tender. Drain. Remove tough center core from giblets. Chop giblets into small pieces. Melt margarine in small skillet. Sauté rice, raisins, giblets, and peanuts until rice and giblets are golden brown. Remove from heat. Add salt and pepper. Add ¼ cup (60 mL) water. Cover and return to heat. Simmer for 15 minutes or until water is absorbed. Remove from heat. Remove cover and allow to cool slightly. Place chicken breast, boned side up between two sheets of plastic wrap or waxed paper. Pound from center with the heel of your hand or edge of a plate to flatten. Place dressing in center. Fold over and secure with toothpicks or poultry pins. Place in small baking dish. Bake in preheated oven at 350° F (175° C) for 1 hour, or until golden brown.

**MICROWAVE:** Sprinkle with paprika and parsley. Cook on High for 18 minutes.

| | |
|---|---|
| **YIELD:** | 1 serving |
| **EXCHANGE:** | 3 ½ lean meat |
| | ½ fruit |
| | ¼ bread |
| | 1 ½ fat |
| **CALORIES:** | 255 |

# El Dorado

| ½ cup | chicken broth | 125 mL |
|---|---|---|
| ½ ounce | fresh oysters | 15 g |
| 1 teaspoon | margarine | 5 mL |
| 1 tablespoon | carrot (grated) | 15 mL |
| 2 tablespoons | celery (chopped) | 30 mL |
| 1 teaspoon | parsley (chopped) | 5 mL |
| 1 ounce | cooked chicken (diced) | 30 g |
| | salt and pepper to taste | |

Heat chicken broth to a boil; add oysters. Cook until edges roll; drain. Heat margarine in heavy skillet. Add carrot, celery, and parsley. Saute until crisp-tender. Add chicken, oysters, and 1 tablespoon (15 mL) of the chicken broth. Cook until thoroughly heated. Drain, if necessary. Add salt and pepper.

**YIELD:** 1 serving
**EXCHANGE:** 1½ lean meat
2 fat
**CALORIES:** 80

# Chicken Livers

| 3 ounces | chicken livers | 90 g |
|---|---|---|
| ½ cup | skim milk | 125 mL |
| 2 tablespoons | flour | 30 mL |
| | salt and pepper to taste | |
| 2 teaspoons | margarine | 10 mL |

Soak chicken livers in skim milk overnight. Drain. Combine flour, salt, and pepper in shaker bag. Add livers, one at a time; shake to coat. Remove livers from bag and shake off excess flour. Melt margarine in small skillet; add livers. Cook until lightly browned and tender.

**YIELD:** 1 serving
**EXCHANGE:** 3 lean meat
2 fat
**CALORIES:** 190

# FISH, SEAFOOD, AND EGGS

## Fish Florentine

| | | |
|---|---|---|
| 2 tablespoons | onion (chopped) | 30 mL |
| ½ cup | mushrooms (chopped) | 125 mL |
| 1 tablespoon | margarine | 15 mL |
| 2 cups | cooked spinach (well drained) | 500 mL |
| 1 teaspoon | lemon juice | 5 mL |
| 1 cup | White Sauce (p. 149) | 250 mL |
| 3 ounces | Cheddar cheese (grated) | 90 g |
| 12 ounces | cooked fish (flaked) | 360 g |

Saute onion and mushrooms in margarine until onion is transparent. Add spinach and lemon juice; mix well. Pour into baking dish or 6 individual baking dishes coated with vegetable cooking spray. Cover with ½ cup (125 mL) of the White Sauce. Sprinkle with 1½ ounces (45 mL) of the cheese. Cover with fish, then with remaining sauce. Sprinkle with remaining cheese. Bake at 350° F (175° C) for 20 minutes.

**MICROWAVE:** Cook on Medium for 10 minutes; turn. Cook 5 minutes more. Hold 3 minutes.

| | |
|---|---|
| **YIELD:** | 6 servings |
| **EXCHANGE 1 SERVING:** | 3½ high-fat meat |
| | 1 vegetable |
| | 1 bread |
| | ½ milk |
| | 1 fat |
| **CALORIES 1 SERVING:** | 215 |

*Note:* Yield is not listed for some recipes where some people are allowed 1 exchange while others are allowed 2 or more.

# Poached Fish

| | | |
|---|---|---|
| 2 pounds | fish (haddock, cod, pollack, salmon) | 1 kg |
| 1 quart | water | 1 L |
| 1 | carrot (sliced) | 1 |
| 1 | onion (sliced) | 1 |
| 1 | bay leaf | 1 |
| ½ teaspoon | thyme | 3 mL |
| ½ teaspoon | whole peppercorns | 3 mL |

Wash fish; wrap in cheesecloth. Combine remaining ingredients in large kettle. Bring to a boil; reduce heat and cook for 15 minutes. Add fish and cook at a simmer. Time depends on thickness, not weight; cook 10 minutes for each inch (2.5 cm) of thickness. Drain in cheesecloth. Turn out onto warm serving platter. Remove skin carefully.

**EXCHANGE 1 OUNCE (30 G):**  1 meat
**CALORIES 1 OUNCES (30 G):**  21

*Note:* Bone is not counted in serving weight.

# Broiled Trout

| | | |
|---|---|---|
| 5-ounce | trout fillet | 150-g |
| 1 teaspoon | margarine | 5 mL |
| dash each | lemon, pepper, marjoram, salt, paprika | |

Clean trout fillet thoroughly; pat dry. Melt margarine; brush on both sides of fillet. Sprinkle with seasonings in order given. Broil 5 to 6 inches (12 to 15 cm) from heat for 10 to 15 minutes. It is not necessary to turn the fillet.

**YIELD:** 1 serving
**EXCHANGE:** 5 lean meat
1 fat
**CALORIES:** 190

# Broiled Smelt

| | | |
|---|---|---|
| 3-ounce | smelt | 90-g |
| | salt and pepper to taste | |
| 1 teaspoon | margarine | 5 mL |
| 1 teaspoon | lemon juice | 5 mL |

Dry smelt thoroughly. Salt and pepper cavity of smelt. Melt margarine; brush on both sides of smelt. Sprinkle with lemon juice. Add salt and pepper. Broil 6 to 8 inches (15 to 20 cm) from heat for 10 to 15 minutes.

**YIELD:** 1 serving
**EXCHANGE:** 3 medium-fat meat
**CALORIES:** 95

# Baked White Fish

| 1 teaspoon | margarine | 5 mL |
| 3-ounce | white fish fillet | 90-g |
| | salt and pepper to taste | |

Melt margarine; brush on both sides of fish fillet. Place fish on aluminum foil. Add salt and pepper. Wrap tightly, securing ends. Place on baking sheet. Bake at 375° F (190° C) for 45 minutes.

**MICROWAVE:** Wrap in plastic wrap; prick wrap. Place on cooking rack. Cook for 7 to 8 minutes, giving package a quarter turn after 4 minutes.

**YIELD:** 1 serving
**EXCHANGE:** 3 medium-fat meat
1 fat
**CALORIES:** 229

# Mustard Halibut Steaks

| 3-ounce | halibut steak | 90 g |
| 1 teaspoon | margarine | 5 mL |
| 1 teaspoon | lemon juice | 5 mL |
| ½ teaspoon | Dijon mustard | 3 mL |
| dash each | lemon rind, sugar replacement | |
| | salt to taste | |

Wash and dry halibut thoroughly. Melt margarine; brush on both sides of halibut. Lay on broiler pan. Brush top with mixture of lemon juice, Dijon mustard, and seasonings. Broil 5 to 6 inches (12 to 15 cm) from heat for 3 to 4 minutes. Turn halibut; repeat on second side.

# Fish Creole

| 2 pounds | whitefish fillets | 1 kg |
|---|---|---|
| 3 cups | water | 750 mL |
| 1 | bay leaf | 1 |
| 3 stalks | celery with tops (chopped) | 3 stalks |
| | salt and pepper to taste | |
| 2 cups | Creole Sauce (p. 143) | 500 mL |

Cut fish into serving pieces. Combine water, bay leaf, celery, salt, and pepper in saucepan. Boil for 2 to 3 minutes. Remove from heat. Add fish pieces and allow water to cool completely. Drain fish and celery; remove bay leaf. Heat Creole Sauce. Add fish and celery. Simmer on low heat for 5 minutes.

YIELD:                              6 servings
EXCHANGE ONE SERVING:   5 medium-fat meat
CALORIES ONE SERVING:   370

# Individual Mackerel

| 3 ounce | cooked mackerel (flaked) | 90 g |
|---|---|---|
| 2 tablespoons | mushrooms (chopped) | 30 mL |
| 1 teaspoon | onion (finely chopped) | 5 mL |
| 1 teaspoon | celery (finely chopped) | 5 mL |
| ½ slice | bread (crumbled) | ½ slice |
| ½ teaspoon | parsley (finely chopped) | 3 mL |
| 1 | egg (beaten) | 1 |
| 1 teaspoon | ketchup | 1 |
| | salt and pepper to taste | |

Combine all ingredients. Mix thoroughly. Place in small baking dish. Bake at 350° F (175° C) for 40 minutes.

**MICROWAVE:** Cook on medium for 10 to 12 minutes.

**YIELD:**     1 serving
**EXCHANGE:** 4 medium-fat meat
            ½ bread
**CALORIES:** 322

# Baked Turbot

| 4-ounce | turbot fillet | 120 g |
|---------|---------------|-------|
| 1 teaspoon | margarine | 5 mL |
| 1 teaspoon | lemon juice | 5 ml |
| dash each | salt, pepper, paprika, parsley | dash each |

Clean turbot fillet thoroughly; pat dry. Melt margarine; brush on both sides of fillet. Place on aluminum foil. Sprinkle with lemon juice, then seasonings. Wrap up fillet securely; lay in cake pan. Bake at 350° F (175° C) for 30 to 40 minutes. Slide fish out of foil onto warm serving plate.

**YIELD:**     1 serving
**EXCHANGE:** 4 medium-fat meat
            1 fat
**CALORIES:** 400

# Salmon Loaf

| | | |
|---|---|---|
| 16 ounces | cooked salmon (flaked) | 500 g |
| 2 tablespoons | onion (chopped) | 30 mL |
| 3 tablespoons | vegetable juice | 45 mL |
| ¼ teaspoon | marjoram | 2 mL |
| 2 | eggs | 2 |
| 1 cup | bread crumbs (finely ground) | 250 mL |
| | salt and pepper to taste | |

If canned salmon is used, drain thoroughly. Combine with remaining ingredients. Blend thoroughly. Allow to rest for 5 minutes, or until bread crumbs are soft. Blend again. Line a 9 x 5-inch (23 x 13-cm) loaf pan with waxed paper. Pack salmon mixture tightly into loaf pan. Bake at 350° F (175° C) for 40 minutes.

**YIELD:** 6 servings
**EXCHANGE 1 SERVING:** 3 medium-fat meat
½ bread
**CALORIES 1 SERVING:** 255

# Cooked Flaked Fish

| | | |
|---|---|---|
| 1 pound | any raw fish | 500g |

Clean fish and cook in salted boiling water for 15 to 20 minutes. Remove skin and bones. Flake fish.

**EXCHANGE 1 OUNCE (30 G) SERVING:** 1 meat
**CALORIES 1 OUNCE (30 G) SERVING:** 25

# Finnan Haddie

| | | |
|---|---|---|
| 3 ounces | cooked finnan haddie | 90 g |
| 1 tablespoon | leek (chopped) | 15 mL |
| 1 tablespoon | green pepper (chopped) | 15 mL |
| 2 teaspoon | pimientos (chopped) | 10 mL |
| ¼ cup | condensed cream of mushroom soup | 60 mL |
| | salt and pepper to taste | |
| ½ ounce | Cheddar cheese (grated) | 15 g |

Arrange finnan haddie in baking dish. Combine leek, green pepper, pimientos, and condensed soup. Stir to mix. Add salt and pepper. Pour over fish. Top with cheese. Bake at 350° F (175° C) for 20 to 25 minutes.

**MICROWAVE:** Cook on Medium for 10 minutes. Turn once.

**YIELD:**    1 serving
**EXCHANGE:** 3½ medium-fat meat
            ½ bread
            1 fat
**CALORIES:** 220

# Great Crab

| | | |
|---|---|---|
| 1 teaspoon | butter | 5 mL |
| dash each | lemon juice, parsley, rosemary, salt, paprika | dash each |
| 2 ounces | crabmeat | 60 g |

Melt butter in small saucepan. Mix in lemon juice and seasonings. Add crabmeat. Toss to coat and heat.

**YIELD:**    1 serving
**EXCHANGE:** 2 lean meat
            1 fat
**CALORIES:** 100

# Marinated Crab Legs

| | | |
|---|---|---|
| ½ cup | Teriyaki Marinade (p. 150) | 125 mL |
| ⅓ cup | lemon juice | 80 mL |
| ½ cup | water | 125 mL |
| 1 teaspoon | basil | 5 mL |
| 1 to 2 pounds | cooked crab legs, shelled | 500 to 1,000 g |

Combine marinade, lemon juice, water, and basil. Add crab legs. (If necessary, add more water to cover legs.) Marinate 2 to 3 hours.

**EXCHANGE 1 OUNCE (30 G):**     1 lean meat
**CALORIES 1 OUNCE (30 G):**     32

# Oysters on the Shell

| | | |
|---|---|---|
| 2 ounce | oysters | 60 g |
| 2 tablespoons | mushroom pieces | 30 mL |
| 1 teaspoon | onion (diced) | 5 mL |
| ¼ cup | vegetable broth | 60 mL |
| 1 slice | bread (finely crumbled) | 1 slice |
| ¼ teaspoon | lemon juice | 1 mL |
| | salt and pepper to taste | |
| 1 | oyster shell | 1 |
| ¼ ounce | Cheddar cheese (grated) | 8 g |

Cook oysters in small amount of boiling salted water until edges start to curl. Drain (reserve some liquid). Combine mushrooms, onion, and broth in saucepan. Bring to a boil. Reduce heat. Add bread crumbs; stir to mix. Remove from heat. Add lemon juice and enough reserved oyster liquid to moisten bread-crumb mixture thoroughly. Add oysters, salt, and pepper. Heap into shell or small baking dish. Top with cheese. Broil until cheese melts.

YIELD: 1 serving
EXCHANGE: 2½ lean meat
1 bread
CALORIES: 125

# Clam Mousse

| 1 envelope | unflavored gelatin | 1 envelope |
|---|---|---|
| 1 cube | vegetable bouillon | 1 cube |
| ½ cup | boiling water | 125 mL |
| 8 ounces | minced clams (and juice) | 240 g |
| 8 ounces | yogurt | 240 g |
| 1 teaspoon | lemon juice | 5 mL |
| 1 teaspoon | celery flakes | 5 mL |
| 1 teaspoon | parsley flakes | 5 mL |
| small dash | cayenne | small dash |

Dissolve gelatin and bouillon cube in boiling water. Beat in remaining ingredients with whisk or electric mixer. Pour into mold and chill until firm.

YIELD: 4 servings
EXCHANGE 1 SERVING: 2 lean meat
¼ milk
CALORIES 1 SERVING: 70

# Shrimp Soufflé

| | | |
|---|---|---|
| 2 ounces | shrimp (canned) | 60 g |
| dash each | thyme, rosemary (crushed), salt, pepper | dash each |
| 1 | egg, separated | 1 |
| | vegetable cooking spray | |

Break shrimp into fine pieces. Add to beaten egg yolk and seasonings. Beat egg whites until stiff. Gently stir half of egg white into shrimp mixture. Gently fold in remaining egg white. Pour into large individual soufflé dish coated with vegetable cooking spray. (Dish should be less than two-thirds full.) Bake at 375° F (190° C) for 15 to 20 minutes.

**YIELD:** 1 serving
**EXCHANGE:** 3 lean meat
**CALORIES:** 205

# Tomato Stuffed with Crab Louis

| | | |
|---|---|---|
| ½ teaspoon | ketchup | 2 mL |
| 1 teaspoon | mayonnaise | 5 mL |
| ¼ teaspoon | Worcestershire sauce | 1 mL |
| 1 ounce | crabmeat | 30 g |
| 1 teaspoon | green onion (finely chopped) | 5 mL |
| 1 tablespoon | celery (finely chopped) | 15 mL |
| 1 tablespoon | green pepper (finely chopped) | 15 mL |
| 1 teaspoon | parsley (finely chopped) | 5 mL |
| 3 | almonds (chopped) | 3 |
| 1 | tomato (peeled) | 1 |
| 1 | lettuce leaf | 1 |

To make Crab Louis, blend ketchup, mayonnaise, and Worcestershire sauce; add crabmeat, green onion, celery, green pepper, parsley, and almonds. Stir to bind; chill. Cut peeled tomato into 7 sections, slicing almost to the bottom. Fill with Crab Louis. Serve on lettuce leaf.

**YIELD:** 1 serving
**EXCHANGE:** 1 medium-fat meat
1 fat
1 vegetable
**CALORIES:** 110

# Venetian Seafood

| | | |
|---|---|---|
| ½ cup | water | 125 mL |
| 2 T. | lime juice | 30 mL |
| 1 T. | chives (finely chopped) | 15 mL |
| 1 t. | garlic powder | 5 mL |
| ½ t. | oregano | 3 mL |
| ½ t. | salt | 3 mL |
| ¼ t. | pepper | 1 mL |
| 1 ounce | fresh or frozen lobster (thawed and cubed) | 30 g |
| 1 ounce | fresh or frozen scallops (thawed) | 30 g |
| 1 ounce | fresh or frozen shrimp (thawed) | 30 g |
| | vegetable cooking spray | |

Make a marinade by blending water, lime juice, and seasonings. Place thawed seafood in deep narrow dish. Pour marinade over seafood to cover. Refrigerate for 3 to 5 hours. (Stir occasionally if seafood is not completely covered with marinade.) Drain. Spray seafood with vegetable cooking spray. Place on baking sheet or dish coated with vegetable cooking spray. Broil 5 to 6 inches (12 to 15 cm) from heat for 5-6 minutes until seafood is tender. Shake baking sheet or dish occasionally to brown seafood evenly.

**YIELD:** 1 serving
**EXCHANGE:** 3 lean meat
**CALORIES:** 90

# Long Island Boil

| | | |
|---|---|---|
| 1 ounce | mussels | 30 g |
| 1 | tomato (peeled and quartered) | 1 |
| 1 | onion (cut into large chunks) | 1 |
| ½ teaspoon | garlic powder | 2 mL |
| 1 teaspoon | parsley | 5 mL |
| 1 ounce | halibut (cut into chunks) | 30 g |
| 1 ounce | scallops | 30 g |
| | salt and pepper to taste | |

Wash mussels thoroughly. Soak in cold water overnight. Steam mussels until shells open; remove mussels from shells. Combine tomato, onion, garlic powder, and parsley. Simmer for 15 minutes. Add halibut and scallops. Cover; simmer 10 minutes. Add mussels, salt and pepper. Heat thoroughly.

**YIELD:** 1 serving
**EXCHANGE:** 3 lean meat
1 vegetable
**CALORIES:** 105

# Lobster Orientale

| | | |
|---|---|---|
| 1 cup | chicken broth | 250 mL |
| 4 | shallots | 4 |
| ¼ teaspoon | ginger | 1 mL |
| ¼ teaspoon | curry powder | 1 mL |
| 1 ounce | pork (cubed) | 30 g |
| 2 ounces | lobster (cubed) | 60 g |
| 1 teaspoon | cornstarch | 5 mL |
| ¼ cup | cold water | 60 mL |
| ½ cup | bean sprouts | 125 mL |

Combine chicken broth, shallots, ginger, and curry powder. Heat to a boil. Add pork; cook until tender. Remove from heat. Add lobster. Dissolve cornstarch in cold water. Combine with pork-lobster mixture. Return to heat; thicken slightly. Add bean sprouts. Heat thoroughly. (Add extra water if mixture thickens too much.)

**YIELD:** 1 serving
**EXCHANGE:** 3 medium-fat meat
**CALORIES:** 140

# Shrimp Creole

| ½ cup | Creole Sauce (p. 143) | 125 mL |
| 10 small | shrimp | 10 |
| 1 cup | rice (cooked) | 250 mL |

Heat Creole Sauce just to a boil. Add shrimp. Remove from heat. Allow to rest 10 minutes. Serve over rice.

**YIELD:** 1 serving
**EXCHANGE:** 2 meat
2 bread
½ vegetable
1 fat
**CALORIES:** 238

# Seafood Medley

| 1 ounce | chunk tuna | 30 g |
| 1 ounce | small shrimp (cooked) | 30 g |
| 1 teaspoon | lemon juice | 5 mL |
| ½ | egg (hard cooked and chopped) | ½ |
| 1 teaspoon | green onion (sliced) | 5 mL |
| 1 | lettuce leaf | 1 |

Combine all ingredients, except lettuce. Chill thoroughly before serving on lettuce leaf with favorite dressing.

YIELD:      1 serving
EXCHANGE:   2½ medium-fat meat
            ¼ vegetable
CALORIES:   137

# Montana Eggs

| 1 | egg (beaten) | 1 |
| ½ ounce | ham (finely chopped) | 15 g |
| 1 teaspoon | onion (finely chopped) | 5 mL |
| | salt and pepper to taste | |
| | vegetable cooking spray | |

Combine egg, ham, onion, salt, and pepper in small bowl. Beat to blend.  Coat pan with vegetable cooking spray; heat to moderately hot. Add egg mixture. Cook on low heat; stir to scramble.

YIELD:      1 serving
EXCHANGE:   1½ high-fat meat
CALORIES:   125

# Basic Omelet

| | vegetable cooking spray | |
| 1 | egg (well beaten) | 1 |
| | salt and pepper to taste | |

Coat pan with vegetable cooking spray; heat pan to moderately hot. Add beaten egg and cook over low heat. Lift edges of egg very carefully to allow uncooked portion of egg to run under. Add salt and pepper. When mixture is firm, fold omelet in half, or roll up jelly-roll style. A filling may be added before folding.

**YIELD:** 1 omelet
**EXCHANGE:** 1 medium-fat meat
**CALORIES:** 78

## Omelet Fillings

Just before folding omelet, add one or more of the following:

*Bean Sprouts:* ¼ cup (60 mL) bean sprouts

*Broccoli:* ¼ cup (60 mL) chopped broccoli

*Cheese:* 1 ounce (30 g) cheese (**EXCHANGE:** 1 high-fat meat; **CALORIES:** 100)

*Chicken Liver:* 1 ounce (30 g) cooked chopped, chicken livers (**EXCHANGE:** 1 lean meat; **CALORIES:** 45)

*Crab:* 1 ounce (30 g) flaked crabmeat (**EXCHANGE:** 1 lean meat; **CALORIES:** 25)

*Dried Beef:* 1 ounce (30 g) chopped dried beef (**EXCHANGE:** 1 medium-fat meat; **CALORIES:** 80)

*Green Pepper and Celery:* 1 tablespoon (15 mL) chopped green pepper, 1 tablespoon (15 mL) chopped celery

*Ham:* 1 ounce (30 g) ham (**EXCHANGE:** 1 high-fat meat; Calories: 100)

*Herbs:* 1 tablespoon (15 mL) chopped parsley, 1 teaspoon (5 mL chives, dash thyme
(Add herbs to beaten egg before cooking.)

*Mushrooms:* 1 tablespoon (15 mL) Mushroom pieces

*Tomato:* 2 tablespoons 30 mL) chopped tomato flesh

*Tuna:*   1 ounce (30 g) drained, water-packed tuna
(**EXCHANGE:** 1 lean meat; **CALORIES:** 50)

*Note:* Where exchange and calories are listed for filling, these must be added to exchange and calories of omelet.

# Eggs Florentine

|                | vegetable cooking spray      |       |
| -------------- | ---------------------------- | ----- |
| 2 tablespoons  | cooked spinach (chopped)     | 30 mL |
| 1              | egg                          | 1     |
|                | salt and pepper to taste     |       |
| ½ ounce        | cheese (grated)              | 15 g  |

Spray individual baking dish with vegetable cooking spray. Cover bottom with spinach. Add egg, salt, and pepper. Top with cheese. Bake at 350° F (175° C) for 15 minutes, or until white is set.

**MICROWAVE:** Prick egg yolk.  Cover. Cook on High for 4 to 5 minutes.

**YIELD:**  1 serving
**EXCHANGE:**  1 ½ medium-fat meat
**CALORIES:** 140

# Cottage Eggs

|         | asparagus spears         | 3    |
| ------- | ------------------------ | ---- |
| 3       | asparagus spears         | 3    |
| 1       | egg                      | 1    |
|         | salt and pepper to taste |      |
| 1 ounce | Swiss cheese (grated)    | 30 g |

Steam asparagus spears until tender. Place in individual baking dish. Poach egg; add salt and pepper. Place on top of asparagus. Top with cheese.  Broil until cheese melts.

**YIELD:** 1 serving
**EXCHANGE:** 2 high-fat meat
1 vegetable
**CALORIES:** 216

# Eggs Benedict

| half | English muffin | half |
|------|----------------|------|
| 1 ounce | lean ham slice | 30 g |
| 1 | egg | 1 |
| 1 tablespoon | Hollandaise Sauce (p. 148-149) | 15 mL |
| | salt and pepper to taste | |

Toast muffin half. Cook ham over low heat. Place on muffin. Poach egg and place on top of ham. Spoon Hollandaise Sauce over egg. Add salt and pepper.

**YIELD:** 1 serving
**EXCHANGE:** 2⅛ high-fat meat
½ bread
1 fat
**CALORIES:** 266

# BREADS

## Bran Bead

| | | |
|---|---|---|
| 3 tablespoons | shortening | 45 mL |
| 3 tablespoons | brown sugar replacement | 45 mL |
| 3 tablespoons | molasses | 45 mL |
| 1 | teaspoon salt | 5 mL |
| ½ cup | bran | 125 mL |
| ¾ cup | boiling water | 190 mL |
| 1 package | dry yeast | 1 pkg. |
| ¼ cup | warm water | 60 mL |
| 2½ cups | flour | 625 mL |
| | Margarine (melted) | |

Place shortening, brown sugar replacement, molasses, salt, and bran in large mixing bowl. Add boiling water. Stir to blend. Soften dry yeast in warm water. Allow to rest for 5 minutes. Add yeast to bran mixture. Add flour, 1 cup (250 mL) at a time, stirring well between additions, until a soft dough is formed. Knead gently for 10 minutes. Shape into loaf. Place in greased 13 x 9 x 2-inch (23 x 13 x 5-cm) loaf pan. Cover; allow to rise for 2 hours. Punch down; allow to rise for 1 hour. Bake at 325° F (165° C) for 50 to 55 minutes. Remove to rack and brush lightly with melted margarine.

YIELD: 1 loaf (14 slices)
EXCHANGE 1 SLICE: 1 bread
CALORIES 1 SLICE: 68

# Jewish Braid Bread (Challah)

| | | |
|---|---|---|
| 1 package | dry yeast | 1 pkg. |
| ¾ cup | warm water | 190 mL |
| 1 teaspoon | salt | 5 mL |
| ¼ cup | ugar replacement | 60 mL |
| 2 tablespoons | margarine (melted) | 30 mL |
| 2 | eggs (well beaten) | 2 |
| 3 cups | flour | 750 mL |
| 1 teaspoon | skim milk | 5 mL |
| | poppy seeds | |

Soften yeast in warm water; allow to rest for 55 minutes. Add salt, sugar replacement, and margarine. Measure 1 tablespoon (15 mL) of the beaten eggs. Place in cup and reserve. Add remaining eggs and 1 cup (250 mL) of the flour to yeast mixture; beat vigorously. Add remaining flour. Turn onto floured board and knead until smooth and elastic. Place in lightly greased bowl; cover. Allow to rise until double in size, about 1½ hours.  Punch down; divide into thirds. Roll into 3 strips, 18-inches (45-cm) long, with the heel of the hand. Braid the 3 strips loosely, tucking under ends. Blend reserved beaten egg with 1 teaspoon (5 mL) skim milk, carefully brush over braid. Sprinkle with poppy seeds; cover. Allow to rise until double in size, about 1½ hours. Bake at 350° F (175° C) for 1 hour, or until done.

**YIELD:**                 1 loaf (18 slices)
**EXCHANGE 1 SLICE:**  1 bread
**CALORIES 1 SLICE:**   70

# Quick Onion Bread

| | | |
|---|---|---|
| 1 loaf | frozen bread dough | 1 loaf |
| 1 package | onion soup mix | 1 package |

Allow bread to thaw as directed on package. Roll dough out on unfloured board. Sprinkle half of soup mix over surface. Roll up jelly-roll style. Knead to work mix into dough; repeat with remaining soup mix. Form into loaf. Place in greased 9 x 5-inch (23 x 13-cm) loaf pan; cover. Allow to rise about 2 hours. Bake at 350° F (175° C) for 30 to 40 minutes, or until done.

**YIELD:** 1 loaf (14 slices)
**EXCHANGE 1 SLICE:** 1 bead
**CALORIES 1 SLICE:** 80

# Apricot Bread

| | | |
|---|---|---|
| 8 | dried apricot halves | 8 |
| ⅓ cup | shortening | 90 mL |
| ¼ cup (packed) | brown sugar replacement | 60 mL (packed) |
| 2 | eggs (beaten) | 2 |
| 1 cup | skim milk | 250 mL |
| ½ teaspoon | salt | 2 mL |
| 1½ teaspoons | baking powder | 7 mL |
| ¼ teaspoon | cinnamon | 1 mL |
| dash | nutmeg | dash |
| ¾ cup | flour | 190 mL |

Soak apricots in warm water for 2 hours. Cook over medium heat for 10 minutes; drain and chop fine. Cream shortening and brown sugar replacement. Add eggs and skim milk; beat thoroughly. Add salt, baking powder, cinnamon, and nutmeg. Stir in apricots and enough of the flour to make a thick cake batter. Pour into greased 9 x 5-inch (23 x

13-cm) loaf pan. Bake at 350° F (175° C) for 1½ hours, or until toothpick comes out clean.

**Microwave:** Bake on Low for 20 minutes. Increase heat to High for 5 minutes, or until toothpick comes out clean. Hold 2 minutes. Turn pan a quarter turn every 10 minutes.

**Yield:** 1 loaf (14 slices)
**Exchange 1 slice:** 1 bread
1 fat
**Calories:** 75

# Raisin Bread

| | | |
|---|---|---|
| 1 package | dry yeast | 1 pkg. |
| ¼ cup | warm water | 60 mL |
| ¾ cups | milk (scaled and cooled) | 180 mL |
| 2 tablespoons | sugar replacement | 30 mL |
| 1 teaspoon | salt | 5 mL |
| 1 | egg | 1 |
| 2 tablespoons | margarine (softened) | 30 mL |
| 3¾ cups | flour | 940 mL |
| 1 cup | raisins | 250 mL |

Soften yeast in warm water; allow to rest for 5 minutes. Combine milk, sugar replacement, salt, egg, and margarine; mix thoroughly. Stir in yeast mixture. Add 1 cup (250 mL) of the flour. Beat until smooth. Mix in raisins. Blend in remaining flour. Knead for 5 minutes. Cover; allow to rise for 2 hours. Punch down; form into loaf. Place in greased 9 x 5-inch (23 x 13-cm) loaf pan; cover. Allow to rise for 1 hour. Bake at 400° F (200° C) for 30 minutes, or until loaf sounds hollow and is golden brown. Remove to rack.

**Yield:** 1 loaf (14 slices)
**Exchange 1 slice:** 1 bread
**Calories 1 slice:** 68

# Pita bread

| | | |
|---|---|---|
| 1 package | dry yeast | 1 pkg. |
| ½ teaspoon | sugar replacement | 3 mL |
| 1 teaspoon | salt | 5 mL |
| 1 tablespoon | liquid shortening | 15 mL |
| 1½ cups | warm water | 375 mL |
| 4 cups | flour | 1,000 mL |

Dissolve yeast, sugar, salt, and liquid shortening in warm water. Add 3 cups (750 mL) of the flour; stir to mix well. (Dough should be fairly stiff; if not, add more flour.) Turn out onto floured surface; knead in remaining flour. (Dough will be very stiff.) Form into 15½-inch (40-cm) tube. Cut into 15 slices. Pat to make circles about 6 inches (15 cm) in diameter. Lay on lightly greased baking pans; cover. Allow to rise until almost doubled, about 1½-2 hours. Bake at 475° F (245° C) for 10 to 12 minutes, or until lightly golden brown, puffed, and hollow. These freeze well.

**YIELD:** 15 pita bread pockets
**EXCHANGE 1 POCKET:** 1½ bread
½ fat
**CALORIES 1 POCKET:** 70

# Pioneer Cornbread

| | | |
|---|---|---|
| 1 | egg | 1 |
| 1 cup | skim milk | 250 mL |
| 2 tablespoons | lo-cal maple syrup | 30 mL |
| 2 tablespoons | margarine (melted) | 30 mL |
| ⅔ cups | cornmeal | 160 mL |
| ¾ cup | flour | 190 mL |
| 1 tablespoon | baking powder | 30 mL |
| 1 teaspoon | salt | 5 mL |

Beat egg until light and lemon colored. Add skim milk, maple syrup, and margarine. Combine cornmeal, flour, baking powder, and salt in large bowl. Stir to blend. Gradually add flour mixture to liquid. Pour into greased 8-inch (20-cm) square pan. Bake at 425° F (220° C) for 20 to 25 minutes.

**MICROWAVE:** Bake on Low for 10 minutes. Increase heat to High for 5 minutes, or until toothpick comes out clean.

**YIELD:** 9 squares
**EXCHANGE 1 SQUARE:** 1½ bread
**CALORIES 1 SQUARE:** 82

# Baking Powder Biscuits

| | | |
|---|---|---|
| 1 cup | flour | 250 mL |
| 1 teaspoon | baking powder | 5 mL |
| ¼ teaspoon | yeast | 2 mL |
| ¼ teaspoon | salt | 2 mL |
| 1 tablespoon | liquid shortening | 15 mL |
| 6 tablespoons | milk | 90 mL |
| | vegetable cooking spray | |

Combine all ingredients, except vegetable cooking spray; mix just until blended. Turn out on floured board. Roll out to a ½-inch (1-cm) thickness. Cut into circles with floured 2-inch (5-cm) cutter. Place on baking sheet coated with vegetable cooking spray; cover. Allow to rest for 10 minutes. Bake at 450° F (230° C) for 12 to 15 minutes, or until lightly browned.

**YIELD:** 10 biscuits
**EXCHANGE 1 BISCUIT:** 1 bread
½ fat
**CALORIES 1 BISCUIT:** 90

# Yeast Rolls

| 1 package | dry yeast | 1 package |
| 1/4 cup | warm water | 60 mL |
| 2 tablespoons | sugar replacement | 30 mL |
| 2 teaspoons | salt | 10 mL |
| 1 tablespoon | margarine (melted) | 15 mL |
| 3/4 cup | warm water | 190 mL |
| 3½ cups | flour | 875 mL |
| 1 | egg (well beaten) | 1 |

Soften yeast in the ¼ cup (60 mL) warm water. Allow to rest for 5 minutes. Combine sugar replacement, salt, margarine, and the ¾ cup (190 mL) warm water; stir to mix. Add 1 cup (250 mL) of the flour; beat well. Blend in yeast mixture and the egg. Add remaining flour; mix well. Knead gently until dough is smooth; cover. Allow to rise for 1 hour. Punch down. Allow to rise for 1 hour. Punch down. Allow to rest for 10 minutes. Shape into 36 rolls. Place on greased cookie sheet or in greased muffin tins. Allow to rise until doubled in size, about 1½-2 hours. Bake at 400° F (200° C) for 20 to 25 minutes, or until golden brown.

**YIELD:**      36 rolls
**EXCHANGE:**      68
**CALORIES 1 ROLL:**   1 bread

# Orange Muffins

| | | |
|---|---|---|
| 1 cup | orange juice | 250 mL |
| 1 tablespoon | orange peel (grated) | 30 mL |
| ½ cup | raisins (soaked) | 125 mL |
| ⅓ cup | sugar replacement | 80 mL |
| 1 tablespoon | margarine | 30 mL |
| 1 | egg | 1 |
| ¼ teaspoon | salt | 2 mL |
| 1 teaspoon | baking soda | 5 mL |
| 1 teaspoon | baking powder | 5 mL |
| ½ teaspoon | vanilla extract | 2 mL |
| 2 cups | flour | 500 mL |

Combine orange juice, orange peel, and raisins. Allow to rest for 1 hour. Cream together the sugar replacement, margarine, and egg. Add salt, baking soda, baking powder, and vanilla extract. Stir in orange juice mixture. Stir in enough of the flour to make a thick cake batter. Spoon into greased muffin tins, filling no more than two-thirds full. Bake at 350° F (175° C) for 20 to 25 minutes, or until done.

**MICROWAVE:** Spoon into 6-ounce (180 mL) custard cups, filling no more than two-thirds full. Cook on Low for 7 to 8 minutes. Increase heat to High for 2 minutes, or until done.

**YIELD:** 24 muffins
**EXCHANGE 1 MUFFIN:** 1 bread
**CALORIES 1 MUFFIN:** 68

# Fresh Apple Muffins

| | | |
|---|---|---|
| 2 tablespoons | soft margarine | 30 mL |
| 2 tablespoons | sugar replacement | 30 mL |
| 1 | egg (beaten) | 1 |
| 1¼ cups | flour | 310 mL |
| ¼ teaspoon | salt | 2 mL |
| 2 teaspoons | baking powder | 10 mL |
| 6 tablespoons | skim milk | 90 mL |
| 1 small | apple (peeled and chopped) | 1 small |

Cream margarine and sugar replacement; add egg. Stir in remaining ingredients. Spoon into greased muffin tins, filling no more than two-thirds full. Bake at 400° F (200° C) for 25 minutes, or until done.

| | |
|---|---|
| **YIELD:** | 12 muffins |
| **EXCHANGE 1 MUFFIN:** | 1 bread |
| **CALORIES 1 MUFFIN:** | 72 |

# Popovers

| | | |
|---|---|---|
| 1 cup | flour | 250 mL |
| ½ teaspoon | salt | 3 mL |
| 2 | eggs | 2 |
| 1 cup | skim milk | 250 mL |

Sift flour and salt together; set aside. Beat eggs and skim milk; add to flour. Beat until smooth and creamy. Pour into heated greased muffin tins, filing half full or less. Bake at 375° F (190° C) for 50 minutes, or until popovers are golden brown and sound hollow. Do not open oven for first 40 minutes.

**YIELD:**                      18 popovers
**EXCHANGE 1 POPOVER:**    ½ bread
                                1/8 meat
**CALORIES 1 POPOVER:**    44

# Soya Crisps

| | | |
|---|---|---|
| 1 cup | soy flour | 250 mL |
| 1 cup | chicken broth | 250 mL |
| 1 tablespoon | liquid shortening | 15 mL |
| 1 teaspoon | salt | 5 mL |

Blend soy flour and broth in saucepan until smooth. Bring gradually to a boil; remove from heat. Blend in liquid shortening and salt. Pour into large flat baking sheet to a depth of no more than ¼ inch (6 mm). Bake at 325° F (165° C) for 30 minutes. Cool slightly. Cut into 2¼-inch (6-cm) squares. Cut diagonally into triangles.

**YIELD:**                      80 chips
**EXCHANGE 10 CHIPS:**    1 lean meat
**CALORIES 10 CHIPS:**    50

# Cake Doughnuts

| | | |
|---|---|---|
| 1 T. | granulated sugar | 15 mL |
| 4 T. | sugar replacement | 60 mL |
| ⅓ cup | buttermilk | 80 mL |
| 1 | egg (well beaten) | 1 |
| 1 cup | flour | 250 mL |
| 1/8 T. | baking soda | 1 mL |
| 1 T. | baking powder | 5 mL |
| dash each | nutmeg, cinnamon, vanilla extract, salt | dash each |
| | oil for deep-fat frying | |

Combine sugars, buttermilk, and egg; beat well. Add remaining ingredients, except oil. Beat just until blended. Heat oil to 375° F (190° C). Drop dough from doughnut dropper into hot fat. Fry until golden brown, turning often. Drain.

**YIELD:** 12 doughnuts
**EXCHANGE 1 DOUGHNUT:** 1 bread
1 fat
**CALORIES 1 DOUGHNUT:** 130

# Tea Scones

| | | |
|---|---|---|
| 1 cup | flour | 250 mL |
| 1 teaspoon | baking powder | 5 mL |
| ¼ teaspoon | salt | 2 mL |
| 1 tablespoon | sugar replacement | 15 mL |
| ¼ cup | margarine (cold) | 60 mL |
| 1 | egg | 1 |
| ¼ cup | evaporated (skim) milk | 60 mL |

Sift flour, baking powder, salt, and sugar replacement. Cut in cold margarine as for pie crust. Beat egg and evaporated milk together thoroughly; stir into flour mixture. Knead gently on lightly floured board. Divide dough in half; roll each half into a circle. Cut circles into quarters. Place on lightly greased cookie sheet. Brush tops with milk. Bake at 450° F (230° C) for 15 minutes, or until done.

**YIELD:** 8 scones
**EXCHANGE 1 SCONE:** 1 bread
**CALORIES 1 SCONE:** 34

## Scone Variations

Stir one of the following into flour mixture for Tea Scones:

*Apple*
8 chopped, dried apple halves
Exchange 1 scone: 1 bread
      ¼ fruit
Calories 1 scone: 44

*Lemon*
1 tablespoon ( 15 mL)grated
    lemon peel
Exchange 1 scone: 1 bread
Calories 1 scone: 34

*Apricot*
8 chopped, dried apricot halves
Exchange 1 scone: 1 bread
      ¼ fruit
Calories 1 scone: 44

*Orange*
1½ tablespoons (25 mL)
grated orange peel
Exchange 1 scone: 1 bread
Calories 1 scone: 34

*Cranberry*
¼ cup (60 mL) chopped
    cranberries
Exchange 1 scone: 1 bread
Calories 1 scone: 34

*Peaches*
8 chopped dried peach halves
Exchange 1 scone: 1 bread
      ½ fruit
Calories 1 scone: 54

*Dates*
8 chopped dates
Exchange 1 scone: 1 bread
    ½ fruit
Calories 1 scone: 54

*Raisin*
4 tablespoons (60 mL) raisins
Exchange 1 scone: 1 bread
      ¼ fruit
Calories 1 scone: 44

# Potato Dumplings

| 1 small | cooked potato | 1 small |
| 1 | egg (beaten) | 1 |
| 2 tablespoons | flour | 30 mL |
| | salt and pepper to taste | |

With a fork, break up and mash the potato. Combine with the remaining ingredients. Beat until light and fluffy. Drop by tablespoonfuls on top of boiling salted water or beef broth. Boil for 5 minutes, or until dumplings rise to surface. Good with Sauerbraten (p. 60).

**YIELD:** 3 or 4 dumplings
**EXCHANGE:** 1 bread
1 meat
**CALORIES:** 140

# Baked Sweet Potato

| ¼ cup | sweet potato or yam (mashed) | 60 mL |
| dash each | salt, pepper, nutmeg | dash each |
| 1 tablespoon | milk | 15 mL |

Combine all ingredients. Beat until smooth and creamy. Bake at 350° F (175° C) for 20 minutes.

**YIELD:** 1 serving
**EXCHANGE:** 1 bread
**CALORIES:** 75

# Mountain Man Pancakes

| 1 | egg | 1 |
| 1¼ cups | buttermilk | 310 mL |
| 1 tablespoon | molasses | 15 mL |
| 2 tablespoons | margarine (melted) | 30 mL |
| 1 cup | flour | 250 mL |
| 1 teaspoon | salt | 5 mL |
| ½ teaspoon | baking soda | 3 mL |
| ½ teaspoon | baking powder | 10 mL |
| ½ cup | yellow cornmeal | 125 mL |
| | vegetable cooking spray | |

Beat egg, buttermilk, molasses, and margarine together until well blended. Add remaining ingredients, except vegetable cooking spray. Stir just enough to blend. Cook in skillet coated with vegetable cooking spray.

**YIELD:** 10 pancakes, 4 inches (9 cm) in diameter each
**EXCHANGE 1 PANCAKE:** 1 bread
1 fat
**CALORIES 1 PANCAKE:** 95

# Potato Pancake

| | | |
|---|---|---|
| 1 medium | raw potato (grated) | 1 medium |
| 1 | egg | 1 |
| 2 | tablespoons flour | 30 mL |
| 2 teaspoons | salt | 10 mL |
| 2 teaspoons | chives | 10 mL |
| | vegetable cooking spray | |

Place grated potato in ice water. Allow to stand for 30 minutes to an hour. Drain; pat potato dry. Place potato in bowl; add egg, flour, salt, and chives. Stir to blend. Divide mixture into 4 parts and spoon into large skillet coated with vegetable cooking spray. Brown on both sides.

**YIELD:** 4 pancakes
**EXCHANGE 2 PANCAKES:** 1 bread
½ medium-fat meat
**CALORIES 2 PANCAKES:** 80

# Potato Puffs

| | | |
|---|---|---|
| ½ cup<br>125 mL | potatoes (cooked and mashed or whipped) | |
| 1 cup | flour | 250 mL |
| 1½ teaspoons | baking powder | 8 mL |
| ½ teaspoon | salt | 3 mL |
| 1 | egg (well beaten) | 3 mL |
| ½ cup | milk | 1 |
| | oil for deep-fat frying | 125 mL |

With a fork, break up and mash enough potatoes to fill a small cup. Combine with remaining ingredients, except oil. Beat well. Heat oil to 375° F (190° C). From tablespoon, drop a walnut-size piece of dough into hot fat. Remove when puff rises to the surface (about 2-3 minutes) and is golden brown. Repeat with remaining dough. Drain.

| | |
|---|---|
| **YIELD:** | 24 puffs |
| **EXCHANGE 2 PUFFS:** | 1 bread |
| | 1½ fat |
| **CALORIES 2 PUFFS:** | 160 |

# Cornbread Stuffing

| | | |
|---|---|---|
| 6 tablespoons | butter | 90 mL |
| 1 large | onion (chopped) | 1 large |
| 1 cup | celery with tops (chopped) | 250 mL |
| 1 teaspoon | thyme | 5 mL |
| 1 teaspoon | sage | 5 mL |
| 1 tablespoon | salt | 15 mL |
| 1 teaspoon | pepper | 5 mL |
| 6 cups | cornbread crumbs | 1.5 L |

Melt butter in medium saucepan. Add onion, celery, thyme, sage, salt, and pepper. Saute over low heat for 3 to 4 minutes. Remove from heat. Add cornbread crumbs; toss to mix. Add water to moisten to stuffing consistency.

| | |
|---|---|
| **YIELD:** | 6 cups (1,500 mL) |
| **EXCHANGE ½ CUP (125 mL):** | 1 bread |
| | 1 fat |
| **CALORIES ½ CUP (125 mL):** | 125 |

# Prune-Apple Stuffing

| | | |
|---|---|---|
| 1 cup | prunes (soaked and chopped) | 250 mL |
| 1½ | cups apples (chopped) | 375 mL |
| ½ cup | raisins | 125 mL |
| 1 teaspoon | cinnamon | 5 mL |
| ½ teaspoon | nutmeg | 3 mL |

Combine fruit and spices; mix thoroughly. Allow to rest for 10 minutes before using.

**YIELD:** 3 cups (750 mL)
**EXCHANGE ¼ CUP (60 mL):** 1 fruit
**CALORIES ¼ CUP (60 mL):** 60

# Herb-Seasoned Stuffing

| | | |
|---|---|---|
| 1-pound | loaf bread (2 to 3 days old) | 500-g loaf |
| ½ cup | butter or margarine | 125 mL |
| 1 teaspoon | thyme | 5 mL |
| 1 teaspoon | sage | 5 mL |
| 1 teaspoon | rosemary | 5 mL |
| 1 teaspoon | dried lemon rind | 5 mL |

Remove crust form bread; cut bread into cubes. Melt butter or margarine in large skillet. Add seasonings; stir to mix. Add bread cubes. Toss or stir lightly to coat bread cubes. Pour onto baking sheet. Allow to dry by air or dry in very slow oven. These dried bread cubes are good as croutons; add salt and water to moisten when ready to use as stuffing.

**YIELD:** 8 cups (2 L)
**EXCHANGE ½ CUP (125 mL):** 1 bread
1 fat
**CALORIES ½ CUP (125 mL):** 75

# Baked Rice

| 1 cube | beef bouillon | 1 cube |
| 1 cup | hot water | 250 mL |
| ¼ cup | rice | 60 mL |
| 1 | green onion (chopped) | 1 |
| 2 tablespoons | celery (chopped) | 30 mL |
| 3 tablespoons | dry bread crumbs | 45 mL |

Dissolve bouillon in hot water. Add rice, green onion, and celery; cover. Cook for 5 minutes. Add bread crumbs. Pour into small baking dish. Bake at 350° F (175° C) for 25 to 30 minutes, or until top is lightly crusted.

**YIELD:** 1 serving
**EXCHANGE:** 1½ bread
**CALORIES:** 115

# Rice Pilaf

| ½ cup | rice | 125 mL |
| 1 teaspoon | butter | 5 mL |
| ½ teaspoon | salt | 3 mL |
| 1 tablespoon | lemon juice | 15 mL |
| 1 cup | boiling water | 250 mL |

Saute rice in butter over low heat in large saucepan. Add remaining ingredients. Bring to a boil. Reduce heat; cover. Simmer until water is absorbed. Fluff with fork before serving.

**YIELD:** 1 cup (250 mL)
**EXCHANGE:** 2 bread
1 fat
**CALORIES:** 150

# Corn Pudding

| | | |
|---|---|---|
| 16-ounce can | corn | 500-g can |
| 1 | egg (beaten) | 1 |
| 1 teaspoon | pimiento (chopped) | 5 mL |
| 1 teaspoon | green pepper | 5 mL |
| 1 teaspoon | margarine (melted) | 5 mL |
| 1 teaspoon | sugar replacement | 5 mL |
| ¾ cup | milk | 180 mL |
| | salt and pepper to taste | |
| | vegetable cooking spray | |

Combine all ingredients, except vegetable cooking spray. Pour into baking dish coated with vegetable cooking spray. Bake at 325° F (163° C) for 35 to 40 minutes, or until firm.

**YIELD:** 6 servings
**EXCHANGE 1 SERVING:** 1 bread
1 fat
**CALORIES 1 SERVING:** 55

# VEGETABLES

## ABC's of Vegetables

| 1 cup | asparagus pieces | 250 mL |
|---|---|---|
| 1 cup | broccoli florets | 250 mL |
| 1 cup | carrot slices | 250 mL |
| 1 cup | spinach (chopped) | 250 mL |
| | vegetable cooking spray | |
| 11-ounce can | condensed cream of mushroom soup | 300-g can |
| 2 tablespoons | onions (finely chopped) | 30 mL |
| 1 teaspoon | thyme | 5 mL |
| ½ cup | water | 125 mL |
| | salt and pepper to taste | |

Layer asparagus, broccoli, carrots, and spinach in a baking dish coated with vegetable cooking spray. Blend remaining ingredients. Pour over vegetables. Cover. Bake at 350° F (175° C) for 30 to 40 minutes, or until vegetables are tender.

**YIELD:** 8 servings
**EXCHANGE 1 SERVING:** 1 vegetable
½ bread
½ fat
**CALORIES 1 SERVING:** 42

# Baked Eggplant

| | | |
|---|---|---|
| 1 slice | eggplant | 1 slice |
| 1 slice | onion | 1 slice |
| 1 ounce | sharp Cheddar cheese (shredded) | 30 g |
| 2 tablespoons | condensed tomato soup | 30 mL |
| 1 teaspoon | dry bread crumbs | 5 mL |
| ¼ teaspoon | thyme | 1 mL |
| ¼ teaspoon | salt | 1 mL |
| | dash pepper dash | |

Cook eggplant and onion in small amount of water until tender. Drain; reserve liquid. Place eggplant and onion in small baking dish. Top with cheese. Blend condensed soup, 1 tablespoon (15 mL) of the eggplant liquid, bread crumbs, thyme, salt, and pepper. Pour over eggplant; cover. Bake at 350° F (175° C) for 30 minutes.

**MICROWAVE:** Uncover. Cook on High for 5 minutes. Turn after 2 minutes.

**YIELD:** 1 serving
**EXCHANGE:** 1 high-fat meat
1 vegetable
**CALORIES:** 161

# Cheese Tomato

| | | |
|---|---|---|
| 1 | tomato (thickly sliced) | 1 |
| | vegetable cooking spray | |
| dash each | celery salt, garlic salt, pepper | dash each |
| 1 ounce | American cheese (grated) | 30 g |

Place tomato slices on broiler pan coated with vegetable cooking spray. Sprinkle with seasonings. Top with cheese. Broil 5 to 6 inches (15 cm) from heat until cheese is melted.

YIELD:        1 serving
EXCHANGE:  1 vegetable
              1 high-fat meat
CALORIES:    140

# Okra and Tomatoes

| | | |
|---|---|---|
| 2 cups | okra | 500 mL |
| ¼ cup | vinegar | 60 mL |
| 2 cups | tomatoes (cut into eighths) | 500 mL |
| 1 cup | onions (coarsely chopped) | 250 mL |
| ½ cup | green pepper (coarsely chopped) | 125 mL |
| sprig | parsley (chopped) | sprig |
| 1 tablespoon | mint (chopped) | 15 mL |
| 1 teaspoon | garlic powder | 5 mL |
| | salt and pepper to taste | |
| | vegetable cooking spray | |

Soak okra in vinegar for 5 minutes. Drain. Pat okra slightly dry. Combine all ingredients (except vinegar) in baking dish coated with vegetable cooking spray. Cover. Bake at 350° F (175° C) for 45 minutes.

YIELD:  5 servings
EXCHANGE 1 SERVING:  1 vegetable
CALORIES 1 SERVING:  31

# Kohlrabi

| | | |
|---|---|---|
| 2 cups | kohlrabi (cut into strips) | 500 mL |
| 2 teaspoons | butter | 10 mL |
| 2 tablespoons | fresh parsley (chopped) | 30 mL |
| | salt and pepper to taste | |

Cook kohlrabi in boiling salted water until soft; drain. Melt butter or margarine in saucepan. Add parsley; sauté over low heat for 2 minutes. Add kohlrabi. Toss to coat. Add salt and pepper.

**YIELD:** 4 servings
**EXCHANGE 1 SERVING:** 1 vegetable
½ fat
**CALORIES 1 SERVING:** 36

# Italian Asparagus

| ½ pound | asparagus spears (cooked or canned) | 250 g |
|---|---|---|
| | vegetable cooking spray | |
| ¼ cup | Tomato Sauce (p. 143) | 60 mL |
| ¼ cup | water | 60 mL |
| ½ teaspoon | oregano | 3 mL |
| ¼ teaspoon | garlic powder | 1 mL |
| | salt and pepper to taste | |
| ¼ cup | Swiss cheese (grated) | 60 mL |

Lay asparagus spears in shallow baking dish coated with vegetable cooking spray. Blend Tomato Sauce, water, oregano, garlic powder, salt, and pepper. Spread evenly over spears. Top with grated cheese. Bake at 350° F (175° C) for 20 to 25 minutes.

**MICROWAVE:** Cook on High for 5 to 6 minutes.

**YIELD:** 4 servings
**EXCHANGE 1 SERVING:** ½ vegetable
½ medium-fat meat
**CALORIES 1 SERVING:** 58

# Cauliflower au Gratin

| | | |
|---|---|---|
| 2 cups | cauliflorets | 500 mL |
| 1 teaspoon | salt | 5 mL |
| 1 teaspoon | butter | 5 mL |
| 1 teaspoon | flour | 5 mL |
| 1 cup | milk (cold) | 250 mL |
| ¼ cup | American cheese (diced) | 60 mL |
| | vegetable cooking spray | |
| | salt and pepper to taste | |

Place cauliflowerets in large kettle. Fill with enough water to cover. Add salt. Bring to a boil; cook 5 minutes. Drain; rinse with cold water. Melt butter or margarine in saucepan. Blend flour with cold milk. Add to melted butter. Cook over low heat, stirring constantly, until slightly thickened. Add cheese; cook until cheese is completely blended. Place cauliflower in baking dish coated with vegetable cooking spray; add salt and pepper. Cover with cheese topping. Bake at 350° F (175° C) for 20 minutes.

YIELD: 4 servings
EXCHANGE 1 SERVING: 1 vegetable
½ medium-fat meat
CALORIES 1 SERVING: 119

# Brussels Sprouts and Mushrooms au Gratin

| | | |
|---|---|---|
| 1 tablespoon | butter | 15 mL |
| 2 cups | Brussels sprouts | 500 mL |
| 1 cup | mushroom pieces | 250 mL |
| | salt and pepper to taste | |
| 2 ounces | Swiss cheese (grated) | 60 g |

Melt butter in skillet. Lightly sauté Brussels sprouts and mushrooms. Add salt and pepper. Remove from heat and pour into baking dish. Cover with cheese. Bake at 350° F (175° C) for 20 to 25 minutes.

**MICROWAVE:** Cook on Medium for 10 minutes. Turn once.

| | |
|---|---|
| **YIELD:** | 4 servings |
| **EXCHANGE 1 SERVING:** | 1 high-fat meat |
| | ½ vegetable |
| **CALORIES 1 SERVING:** | 65 |

# Baked Vegetable Medley

| | | |
|---|---|---|
| 1 cup | 2-inch (5-cm) cubes eggplant | 250 mL |
| 1 cup | 2-inch (5-cm) slices okra | 250 mL |
| 1 cup | bean sprouts | 250 mL |
| ½ cup | small mushrooms | 125 mL |
| 1 | onion (cut into eighths) | 1 |
| | vegetable cooking spray | |
| 11-ounce can | condensed cream of celery soup | 300-g can |
| ¼ cup | water | 60 mL |
| | salt and pepper to taste | |
| 1 slice | bread (finely crumbled) | 1 slice |

Combine all vegetables in baking dish coated with vegetable cooking spray  Blend condensed soup and water; add salt and pepper. Pour over vegetables. Top with bread crumbs. Cook at 325° F (165° C) for 25 to 30 minutes, or until hot, and crumbs are golden brown.

| | |
|---|---|
| **YIELD:** | 8 servings |
| **EXCHANGE 1 SERVING:** | 1 vegetable |
| | ½ bread |
| **CALORIES 1 SERVING:** | 49 |

# Shredded Cabbage

| 1 head | cabbage (coarsely shredded) | 1 head |
| 2 teaspoons | butter | 10 mL |
| ½ teaspoon | nutmeg | 2 mL |
| | salt and pepper to taste | |

Cook cabbage in a small amount of boiling salted water until tender; drain. Press out excess moisture or pat dry. Melt butter in skillet. Add nutmeg; stir to blend. Add cabbage; toss to coat. Add salt and pepper.

**YIELD:** 4 servings
**EXCHANGE 1 SERVING:** ½ vegetable
½ fat
**CALORIES 1 SERVING:** 32


# Irish Vegetables

| 1 | bay leaf | 1 |
| 1 cup | water | 250 mL |
| 2 tablespoons | wine vinegar | 30 mL |
| ½ cup | corn | 125 mL |
| ½ cup | celery (sliced) | 125 mL |
| ½ cup | broccoli florets | 125 mL |
| ½ cup | carrot (sliced) | 125 mL |
| ½ cup | cauliflorets | 125 mL |
| ¼ cup | pimiento (chopped) | 60 mL |
| | salt and pepper to taste | |

Combine bay leaf, water, and wine vinegar in medium saucepan. Bring to a boil; add vegetables. Simmer until vegetables are tender. Drain; remove bay leaf. Add salt and pepper.

| **YIELD:** | 5 servings |
|---|---|
| **EXCHANGE 1 SERVING:** | 1 bread |
| **CALORIES 1 SERVING:** | 51 |

# Spiced Bean Sprouts

| 2 cups | bean sprouts | 500 mL |
|---|---|---|
| ½ teaspoon | caraway seeds | 2 mL |
| ½ teaspoon | basil | 2 mL |
| 2 teaspoons | butter | 10 mL |
| | salt and pepper to taste | |

Combine bean sprouts, caraway seeds, and basil in saucepan with small amount of water. Cook until hot and tender; drain. Place in serving dish; top with butter, salt, and pepper. Toss to coat.

| **YIELD:** | 4 servings |
|---|---|
| **EXCHANGE 1 SERVING:** | ¼ vegetable |
| | ½ fat |
| **CALORIES 1 SERVING:** | 25 |

# German Green Beans

| 2 cups | green beans | 500 mL |
|---|---|---|
| 1 slice | bacon | 1 slice |
| ¼ cup | onion (chopped) | 60 mL |
| 1 teaspoon | flour | 5 mL |
| ¼ cup | vinegar | 60 mL |
| ½ cup | water | 125 mL |
| 2 tablespoons | sugar replacement | 30 mL |

Cook green beans in boiling salted water until tender; drain. Cut bacon into ½-inch (12-mm) pieces. Place in skillet; add onion. Saute until bacon is crisp and onion is tender; drain. Blend flour, vinegar, water, and sugar replacement in screw-top jar. Pour over bacon and onion. Cook over low heat to thicken slightly. Add green beans.

| | |
|---|---|
| **YIELD:** | 4 servings |
| **EXCHANGE 1 SERVING:** | ½ vegetable |
| | ¼ bread |
| | ½ fat |
| **CALORIES 1 SERVING:** | 52 |

# Pizza Beans

| | | |
|---|---|---|
| 2 cups | green beans | 500 mL |
| 1 tablespoon | lemon juice | 15 mL |
| ¼ teaspoon | oregano | 1 mL |
| 1 teaspoon | pimiento (chopped) | 5 mL |
| dash each | garlic powder, salt | dash each |

Cook green beans in boiling salted water until tender; drain. Combine lemon juice, oregano, pimiento, garlic powder, and salt. Pour over beans; toss.

| | |
|---|---|
| **YIELD:** | 5 servings |
| **EXCHANGE 1 SERVING:** | 1 vegetable |
| **CALORIES 1 SERVING:** | 32 |

# Whipped Summer Squash

| | | |
|---|---|---|
| 3 cups | summer squash | 750 mL |
| ¼ cup | evaporated milk | 60 mL |
| 2 teaspoons | butter | 10 mL |
| | salt and pepper to taste | |

Peel and cut squash into small pieces. Place in saucepan with small amount of water. Bring to a boil; reduce heat and simmer until squash is crisp-tender. Drain. Beat squash with rotary beater; add evaporated milk and butter. Beat until light and fluffy. Add salt and pepper.

| | |
|---|---|
| **YIELD:** | 4 servings |
| **EXCHANGE 1 SERVING:** | 1 vegetable |
| | 1 fat |
| **CALORIES 1 SERVING:** | 68 |

# Spiced Beets

| | | |
|---|---|---|
| ½ cup | wine vinegar | 125 mL |
| ¼ cup | water | 60 mL |
| 1 | bay leaf | 1 |
| 1 | whole clove | 1 |
| 1 teaspoon | black pepper | 5 mL |
| 3 tablespoons | sugar replacement | 45 mL |
| 2 cups | beets (sliced) | 500 mL |

Combine all ingredients except beets. Bring to a boil. Add beets; simmer for 10 minutes, or until tender.

**MICROWAVE:** Combine all ingredients, except beets. Cook on High for 2 minutes. Add beets. Cook on Medium for 2 minutes.

| | |
|---|---|
| **YIELD:** | 4 servings |
| **EXCHANGE 1 SERVING:** | 1 bread |
| **CALORIES 1 SERVING:** | 36 |

# Indian Squash

| | | |
|---|---|---|
| 2 cups | acorn squash (cubed) | 500 mL |
| 2 teaspoons | margarine | 10 mL |
| 1 teaspoon | orange rind | 5 mL |
| ¼ cup | orange juice | 60 mL |
| 2 tablespoons | sugar replacement | 30 mL |

Cook squash in small amount of boiling water until crisp-tender; drain. Melt margarine in saucepan. Add orange rind, juice, and sugar replacement. Cook over low heat until sugar is dissolved. Add squash; cover Continue cooking until squash is tender.

| | |
|---|---|
| **YIELD:** | 4 servings |
| **EXCHANGE 1 SERVING:** | 1 bread |
| | ½ fat |
| **CALORIES 1 SERVING:** | 60 |

# Beans Orientale

| | | |
|---|---|---|
| 1½ cups | French-cut green beans (cooked) | 375 mL |
| 2 tablespoons | almonds (blanched and slivered) | 30 mL |
| ½ cup | mushroom pieces | 125 mL |
| 2 teaspoons | butter | 10 mL |
| | salt and pepper to taste | |

Heat green beans; drain. Sauté almonds and mushrooms in butter. Add green beans. Add salt and pepper.

**MICROWAVE:** Melt butter in bowl. Add almonds and mushrooms. Cover. Cook on High for 30 seconds. Add green beans. Cook on Medium for 2 to 3 minutes.

| **YIELD:** | 4 servings |
| **EXCHANGE 1 SERVING:** | ½ vegetable |
| | ½ fat |
| **CALORIES 1 SERVING:** | 45 |

# Vegetable Casserole

| | | |
|---|---|---|
| 1 cup | peas | 250 mL |
| 1 cup | green beans | 250 mL |
| 1 cup | carrots (sliced) | 250 mL |
| 1 cup | mushrooms | 250 mL |
| 1 | egg | 1 |
| 1 teaspoon | margarine (melted) | 5 mL |
| ½ cup | milk | 125 mL |
| | salt and pepper to taste | |
| | vegetable cooking spray | |

Cook vegetables in small amount of boiling salted water until crisp-tender; drain. Chop vegetables fine. Whip egg until lemon colored; add margarine and milk. Blend well. Add chopped vegetables, salt, and pepper. Pour into baking dish coated with vegetable cooking spray. Cover. Bake at 350° F (175° C) for 45 minutes, or until set.

| **YIELD:** | 8 servings |
| **EXCHANGE 1 SERVING:** | 1 vegetable |
| **CALORIES 1 SERVING:** | 36 |

# Pea Pod-Carrot Sauté

| | | |
|---|---|---|
| 1 cup | pea pods | 250 mL |
| 1 cup | carrots (sliced) | 250 mL |
| 1 teaspoon | salt | 5 mL |
| 2 teaspoons | margarine | 10 mL |
| 1 tablespoon | Worcestershire sauce | 15 mL |

Combine pea pods and carrots in saucepan. Cover with water; add salt. Cook until tender; drain. Melt margarine in saucepan. Add Worcestershire sauce; stir to blend. Add pea pods and carrots. Toss to cat.

| | |
|---|---|
| **YIELD:** | 4 servings |
| **EXCHANGE 1 SERVING:** | ½ bread |
| | ½ fat |
| **CALORIES 1 SERVING:** | 50 |

# Circus Carrots

| | | |
|---|---|---|
| 2 cups | carrots (finger or julienne cut) | 500 mL |
| 2 teaspoons | butter | 10 mL |
| 2 tablespoons | lemon juice | 30 mL |
| 2 teaspoons | parsley flakes | 10 mL |

Cook carrots in boiling salted water until tender; keep warm. Melt butter; add lemon juice and parsley flakes. Add warm carrots; toss to coat.

**MICROWAVE:** Cook carrots in small amount of water on High for 2 minutes. Drain. Add remaining ingredients. Cover. Cook on High for 2 minutes. Toss to mix.

| | |
|---|---|
| **YIELD:** | 4 servings |
| **EXCHANGE 1 SERVING:** | ¼ fat |
| | 1 bread |
| **CALORIES 1 SERVING:** | 59 |

# Candied Carrot Squares

| 4 | carrots | 4 |
|---|---|---|
| 1 teaspoon | salt | 5 mL |
| 2 tablespoons | brown sugar replacement | 30 mL |
| 2 teaspoons | butter | 10 mL |
| ½ cup | lo-cal cream soda (or any white) | 125 mL |

Cut carrots into lengths to make squares. Place carrots in saucepan and cover with water; add salt. Cook until crisp-tender; drain. Place in baking dish. Sprinkle carrots with brown sugar replacement; dot with butter; add white soda. Bake at 350° F (175° C) for 30 minutes. Turn carrots gently two or three times during baking.

| | |
|---|---|
| **YIELD:** | 4 servings |
| **EXCHANGE 1 SERVING:** | 1 bread |
| | ½ fat |
| **CALORIES 1 SERVING:** | 47 |

# Spinach with Onion

| 2 pounds | fresh spinach | 1 kg |
|---|---|---|
| 2 teaspoons | margarine | 10 mL |
| ½ cup | onion (sliced) | 125 mL |
| dash each | nutmeg, thyme, salt, pepper | dash each |

Rinse spinach thoroughly; place in top of double boiler and heat until wilted. Drain and chop coarsely. Melt margarine in skillet; add onion. Sauté over high heat until onion is brown on the edges. Add seasonings. Stir to blend. Add spinach and toss to blend.

| | |
|---|---|
| **YIELD:** | 4 servings |
| **EXCHANGE 1 SERVING:** | ½ vegetable |
| | ½ fat |
| **CALORIES 1 SERVING:** | 37 |

# Zucchini Florentine

| | | |
|---|---|---|
| 4 small | zucchini | 4 small |
| 2 teaspoons | margarine | 10 mL |
| 1 cup | fresh spinach (chopped) | 250 mL |
| 1 cup | skim milk | 250 mL |
| 3 | eggs (slightly beaten) | 3 |
| 1 teaspoon | salt | 5 mL |
| ¼ teaspoon | pepper | 1 mL |
| ¼ teaspoon | thyme | 1 mL |
| ¼ teaspoon | paprika | 1mL |

Cut zucchini into thin slices. Melt margarine in baking dish; add zucchini. Bake at 400° F (200° C) for 15 minutes. Add spinach. Blend skim milk, eggs, salt, pepper, and thyme. Pour over vegetables. Sprinkle with paprika. Bake at 350° F (175° C) for 40 minutes, or until set.

**YIELD:** 6 servings
**EXCHANGE 1 SERVING:** 1 vegetable
½ high-fat meat
**CALORIES 1 SERVING:** 82

# Zucchini Wedges

| | | |
|---|---|---|
| 4 small | zucchini | 4 small |
| 2 teaspoons | margarine | 10 mL |
| 2 teaspoons | onion (grated) | 10 mL |
| 1 cube | beef bouillon | 1 cube |
| 2 tablespoons | boiling water | 30 mL |

Cut zucchini in half lengthwise. Melt margarine in skillet. Add onion and bouillon cube. Press bouillon cube against bottom of skillet to crush. Stir to blend. Place zucchini cut side down in skillet. Sauté until golden brown; turn. Add boiling water; cover. Cook over low heat for 10 minutes, or until tender.

**YIELD:** 4 servings
**EXCHANGE 1 SERVING:** ½ vegetable
½ fat
**CALORIES 1 SERVING:** 37

# SALADS

## Perfect Salad

| | | |
|---|---|---|
| ½ envelope | unflavored gelatin | ½ env. |
| ¼ cup | cold water | 60 mL |
| 1 tablespoon | sugar replacement | 15 mL |
| ½ teaspoon | salt | 2 mL |
| ¾ cup | hot water | 180 mL |
| 1 tablespoon | lemon juice | 15 mL |
| 2 | cucumbers (grated) | 2 |
| ¼ cup | carrot (grated) | 60 mL |
| ¼ cup | onion (chopped) | 60 mL |
| 3 ounces | cream cheese | 90 g |
| 2 tablespoons | lo-cal mayonnaise | 30 mL |

Dissolve gelatin in cold water. Add gelatin mixture, sugar replacement, and salt to hot water; stir until dissolved. Add lemon juice, cucumbers, carrot, and onion. Beat cream cheese with mayonnaise until smooth. Blend into vegetable mixture. Pour into mold and chill.

| | |
|---|---|
| YIELD: | 8 servings |
| EXCHANGE 1 SERVING: | ½ vegetable |
| | 1 fat |
| CALORIES 1 SERVING: | 73 |

# Mushroom Salad

| | | |
|---|---|---|
| ½ head | iceberg lettuce | ½ head |
| ½ head | Boston lettuce | ½ head |
| 1 | cucumber | 1 |
| ½ pound | green beans | 250 g |
| ½ pound | mushrooms | 250 g |
| ¼ cup | lo-cal French dressing | 60 mL |

Rinse lettuce. Break into large pieces. Peel and slice cucumber into ¼-inch (6-mm) slices. Rinse green beans; cut beans into 1-inch (2.5-cm) pieces. Place greens, cucumber, and beans into plastic bag or tightly covered container. Store in refrigerator 4 to 6 hours or overnight to crisp. Trim mushroom stems to ¼-inch (6-mm) of cap. (Peel mushrooms if discolored.) Cut mushrooms in thin slices. Just before serving, carefully pat greens, cucumber, and beans dry on towel. Place in wooden bowl; cover with French dressing. Toss to lightly coat all ingredients with dressing. Top with mushrooms.

**YIELD:** 8 servings
**EXCHANGE 1 SERVING:** 1 vegetable
**CALORIES 1 SERVING:** 60

# Chinese Salad

| | | |
|---|---|---|
| 1 head | Bibb lettuce | 1 head |
| 1 head | Boston lettuce | 1 head |
| 2 stalks | Chinese cabbage | 2 stalks |
| 8-ounce can | water chestnuts | 225-g can |
| 8-ounce can | bamboo shoots | 225-g can |
| 1 cup | bean sprouts | 250 mL |
| ½ cup | Soy French Dressing (p. 145) | 125 mL |

Rinse lettuce and cabbage leaves. Break into bite-size pieces. Place in plastic bag or tightly covered container. Store in refrigerator 4 to 6 hours or overnight to crisp. Drain water chestnuts, bamboo shoots, and bean sprouts. Rinse with cold water. Drain thoroughly. Thinly slice the water chestnuts. Carefully pat greens dry with towel. Place in wooden bowl. Top with water chestnuts, bamboo shoots, and bean sprouts. Cover with Soy French Dressing. Toss lightly until all ingredients are coated.

| | |
|---|---|
| **YIELD:** | 12 servings |
| **EXCHANGE 1 SERVING:** | ½ vegetable |
| **CALORIES 1 SERVING:** | 40 |

# Dandelion Salad

| | | |
|---|---|---|
| 1 cup | young dandelion greens | 250 mL |
| 1 head | iceberg lettuce | 1 head |
| 2 tablespoons | lo-cal Italian dressing | 30 mL |
| 2 | tomatoes | 2 |
| 1 small | cucumber | 1 small |
| 2 tablespoons | lo-cal bleu cheese dressing | 30 mL |
| 1 tablespoon | skim milk | 15 mL |

Rinse greens and lettuce. Pat dry with towel. Break into large pieces. Place in large plastic bag. Sprinkle with Italian dressing. Close tightly and store in refrigerator to crisp. Shake occasionally. Peel tomatoes and remove seeds; slice tomato flesh into strips. Peel cucumber; slice into ⅛-inch (3-mm) slices. Place greens, lettuce, tomatoes, and cucumber in wooden bowl. Blend bleu cheese dressing with skim milk. Cover salad with dressing. Toss to coat all ingredients.

YIELD: 6 servings
EXCHANGE 1 SERVING: Negligible
CALORIES 1 SERVING: Negligible

*Added Touch:* Top each serving with a few Garlic Croutons (p. 15). Add exchange and calories for croutons.

# Jean's Vegetable Salad

| | | |
|---|---|---|
| 1 cup | asparagus, cut into 2-inch (5-cm) pieces | 250 mL |
| 1 cup | broccoli florets | 250 mL |
| 1 cup | cauliflorets | 250 mL |
| ½ cup | celery (sliced) | 125 mL |
| ½ cup | cucumber (scored and sliced) | 125 mL |
| 1 cup | fresh mushrooms (sliced) | 250 mL |
| 1 cup | green pepper (sliced) | 250 mL |
| ½ cup | radishes (sliced) | 125 mL |
| 10 | pitted black olives (sliced) | 10 |
| ½ cup | lo-cal Italian dressing | 125 mL |

Combine all vegetables in large bowl. Cover with Italian dressing. Marinate overnight. Toss frequently.

YIELD: 7 servings
EXCHANGE 1 SERVING: 1 vegetable
CALORIES 1 SERVING: 45

# Radish Salad

| | | |
|---|---|---|
| 1 teaspoon | salt | 5 mL |
| 1 teaspoon | garlic powder | 5 mL |
| 1 teaspoon | Dijon mustard | 5 mL |
| 1 tablespoon | wine vinegar | 15 mL |
| 2 tablespoons | liquid shortening | 30 mL |
| 2 teaspoons | lemon juice | 10 mL |
| 1 | watercress (small bunch) | 1 |
| ½ head | iceberg lettuce | ½ head |
| 1 bunch | red radishes | 1 bunch |

Combine salt, garlic powder, Dijon mustard, vinegar, liquid shortening, and lemon juice in screw top jar. Shake to blend. Coarsely chop watercress, lettuce and radishes; place in salad bowl. Add dressing; toss to blend.

**YIELD:** 6 servings
**EXCHANGE 1 SERVING:** 1 fat
**CALORIES 1 SERVING:** 60

# Maude's Green Salad

| | | |
|---|---|---|
| ½ head | iceberg lettuce | ½ head |
| ½ head | Boston lettuce | ½ head |
| ½ head | chicory | ½ head |
| ½ pound | spinach | 250 g |
| ½ head | romaine lettuce | ½ head |
| 5 tablespoons | lo-cal Italian dressing | 75 mL |
| 1 tablespoon | Parmesan cheese | 15 mL |

Rinse and crisp the salad greens. Break iceberg lettuce into bite-size pieces. Carefully pat iceberg dry on towel. Place in large plastic bag. Add 1 tablespoon (15 mL) Italian dressing. Shake lightly until all leaves are covered. Place in strip on medium platter or plate. Repeat with each green. Sprinkle lightly with Parmesan cheese.

YIELD: 10 servings
EXCHANGE: Negligible
CALORIES: Negligible

# German Potato Salad

| | | |
|---|---|---|
| 6 slices | bacon (crispy fried) | 6 slices |
| 1½ cups | cold water | 375 mL |
| 3 tablespoons | flour | 45 mL |
| 1 medium | onion (chopped) | 1 medium |
| 3 tablespoons | sugar replacement | 45 mL |
| ¼ cup | vinegar | 60 mL |
| 6 medium | boiled potatoes (sliced) | 6 medium |

Remove excess grease from bacon with paper towel. Break bacon into small pieces. Blend cold water and flour. Pour into saucepan. Add onion, sugar replacement, and vinegar. Heat, stirring, until thickened. Add bacon and potatoes while still warm from boiling and frying.

YIELD: 8 servings
EXCHANGE 1 SERVING: 1 bread
1 fat
CALORIES 1 SERVING: 113

# Swiss Salad

| | | |
|---|---|---|
| 1 small head | iceberg lettuce | 1 small head |
| 1 head | romaine lettuce | 1 head |
| ¼ pound | fresh spinach | 125 g |
| 1 large | cucumber | 1 large |
| 1 | green pepper | 1 |
| 1 cup | cherry tomatoes | 250 mL |
| ½ cup | lo-cal French dressing | 125 mL |

Rinse and wash greens. Drain thoroughly. Break into large pieces; place in plastic bag or tightly covered container. Store in refrigerator 4 to 6 hours or overnight to crisp. Score cucumber with tines of fork. Cut into ⅛-inch (3-mm) slices. Cut green pepper into thin rings. Cut cherry tomatoes in half. Just before serving, carefully pat greens dry on towel. Place greens in large wooden bowl; cover with French dressing. Toss greens lightly, coating all leaves with dressing. Top with cucumber, green pepper, and cherry tomatoes. Serve immediately.

**YIELD:**                 16 servings
**EXCHANGE 1 SERVING:**  ½ vegetable
**CALORIES 1 SERVING:**    32

# Marinated Cucumbers

| | | |
|---|---|---|
| 2 to 3 | cucumbers (large) | 2 to 3 |
| 1 teaspoon | salt | 5 mL |
| 1 teaspoon | sugar replacement | 5mL |
| ¼ cup | vinegar | 60 mL |
| ⅛ teaspoon | pepper | 1 mL |

Score cucumbers with tines of fork. Cut into very thin slices. Sprinkle with salt. Chill 2 hours; drain well. Sprinkle with sugar replacement; add vinegar and pepper. Marinate 30 minutes or more before serving.

**YIELD:**     6 to 8 servings
**EXCHANGE:**  Negligible
**CALORIES:**  Negligible

# Asparagus Salad

| | | |
|---|---|---|
| ¼ pound | spinach | 125 g |
| 1 head | romaine lettuce | 1 head |
| 10 spears | raw asparagus | 10 spears |
| ½ head | red cabbage | ½ head |
| ½ cup | celery (sliced) | 125 mL |
| ½ | cucumber (peeled and sliced) | ½ |
| ½ cup | Lemon French Dressing (p. 145) | 125 mL |

Rinse greens. Break into bite-size pieces. Place in plastic bag or tightly covered container. Store in refrigerator 4 to 6 hours or overnight to crisp. Wash asparagus spears and cut into 2-inch (5-cm) pieces. Shred cabbage as for coleslaw; remove all hard pieces. Just before serving, carefully pat greens dry on towel. Place all ingredients in wooden bowl. Toss lightly to coat all ingredients with Lemon French Dressing.

**YIELD:** 12 servings
**EXCHANGE 1 SERVING:** ½ vegetable
**CALORIES 1 SERVING:** 42

# Hot Green Pepper Salad

| | | |
|---|---|---|
| 4 | green peppers | 4 |
| 1 tablespoon | butter | 15 mL |
| 1 teaspoon | oregano | 5 mL |
| ½ teaspoon | thyme | 2 mL |
| | salt and pepper to taste | |
| ½ cup | mushroom pieces | 125 mL |

Rinse green peppers. Cut them into quarters. Melt butter in skillet. Add seasonings, green peppers, and mushrooms. Cook over low heat for 10 minutes. Serve immediately.

**YIELD:** 4 servings
**EXCHANGE 1 SERVING:** 1 vegetable
1 fat
**CALORIES 1 SERVING:** 60

# Shrimp and Green Bean Salad

| 2 cups | green beans | 500 mL |
| 2 cups | shrimp | 500 mL |
| ½ cup | mushrooms (thinly sliced) | 125 mL |
| ¼ cup | Bay Salad Dressing (p. 147) | 60 mL |
| | lettuce leaves | |

Rinse and snap green beans. Cook in small amount of boiling salted water until crisp-tender. Drain and cool immediately in ice water; chill. Clean and devein shrimp, or use canned shrimp. Rinse thoroughly under cold water; chill. Combine green beans, shrimp, and mushrooms in bowl. Sprinkle with Bay Salad Dressing. Toss to coat. Chill thoroughly before serving. Serve on lettuce leaves.

**YIELD:** 4 servings
**EXCHANGE 1 SERVING:** 1 lean meat
½ vegetable
**CALORIES 1 SERVING:** 62

# Salmon Salad Plate

| | | |
|---|---|---|
| 1 ounce | cold salmon (cooked) | 30 g |
| ½ small | tomato | ½ small |
| ¼ cup | carrot sticks | 60 mL |
| ¼ | green pepper (sliced) | ¼ |
| ¼ cup | eggplant sticks | 60 mL |
| 1 | egg (hard cooked) | 1 |
| 1 tablespoon | cottage cheese | 15 mL |
| | salt and pepper to taste | |
| | lettuce leaf | |

Chill salmon. Peel tomato and remove seeds; slice tomato flesh into strips. Cook carrot, green pepper, eggplant, and tomato in boiling salted water until crisp-tender. (Remember, the carrot sticks may take more time to cook than the other vegetables.) Drain and chill. Cut egg in half lengthwise. Mash egg yolk with cottage cheese, salt, and pepper; stuff egg white halves. Arrange cooked salmon, vegetables, and stuffed eggs on crisp lettuce leaf.

**YIELD:** 1 serving
**EXCHANGE:** 2⅓ lean meat
1 vegetable
**CALORIES:** 193

# Waldorf Salad

| | | |
|---|---|---|
| 1 cup | celery (sliced) | 250 mL |
| 1 cup | seedless green grapes (halved) | 250 mL |
| 1 cup | apple (diced) | 250 mL |
| 4 | dates (pitted and thinly sliced) | 4 |
| ½ cup | walnuts (chopped) | 125 mL |
| ¼ cup | mayonnaise | 60 mL |
| 2 tablespoons | dry white wine | 30 mL |
| | lettuce leaves | |

Place celery, grapes, apple, dates, and walnuts into bowl. Blend mayonnaise with wine; pour into bowl. Stir to blend with celery, fruit and walnuts. Use slotted serving spoon to serve, shaking spoon slightly to remove excess dressing. Serve on crisp lettuce leaves.

| | |
|---|---|
| **YIELD:** | 7 servings |
| **EXCHANGE 1 SERVING:** | 2 fruit |
| | ¼ vegetable |
| | 1 fat |
| **CALORIES 1 SERVING:** | 105 |

# Herring Salad Plate

| | | |
|---|---|---|
| 1 ounce | salted herring | 30 g |
| ½ small | onion (thinly sliced) | ½ small |
| ¼ cup | beets (sliced) | 60 mL |
| | Italian or French dressing | |
| | Lettuce leaf | |

Soak herring overnight in water. Remove skin and bones. Cut into 1-inch (2.5-cm) pieces. Place herring, onion, and beets in glass bowl. Cover with dressing. Marinate 4 to 5 hours or overnight. Drain. (Keep liquid; it makes a very good salad dressing.) Arrange herring, onion, and beets on crisp lettuce leaf.

| | |
|---|---|
| **YIELD:** | 2 servings |
| **EXCHANGE 1 SERVING:** | ½ lean meat |
| | 1 bread |
| **CALORIES 1 SERVING:** | 50 |

# Lime Avocado Salad

| 1 package | (⅝ ounce) lo-cal lime gelatin (both envelopes) | 1 package (20 g) |
|---|---|---|
| 1½ cups | boiling water | 375 mL |
| 3 ounces | cream cheese | 90 g |
| ½ cup | lo-cal whipped topping (prepared) | 125 mL |
| ½ cup | avocado (cubed) | 125 mL |
| ½ cup | unsweetened fruit cocktail | 125 mL |
| | vegetable cooking spray | |
| | shredded lettuce | |

Dissolve gelatin in boiling water. Cool to consistency of beaten egg whites. Beat cream cheese; blend into gelatin mixture. Fold prepared whipped topping into gelatin mixture. Chill until quite firm. Fold in avocado and fruit cocktail. Pour into 1-quart (1-L) ring mold coated with vegetable cooking spray. Chill until set. Serve on bed of shredded lettuce.

**YIELD:** 8 servings
**EXCHANGE 1 SERVING:** ½ vegetable
½ lean meat
1 fat
**CALORIES 1 SERVING:** 78

# Cantaloupe Bowl

| 4 | strawberries | 4 |
|---|---|---|
| 4 | fresh pineapple cubes | 4 |
| 1 teaspoon | sugar replacement | 5 mL |
| ¼ | 6-inch (15-cm) cantaloupe | ¼ |

Sprinkle strawberries and pineapple with sugar replacement. Fill hollow of cantaloupe with fruit mixture.

# Grapefruit Salad

| ¼ cup | cranberries | 60 mL |
| 1½ cups | grapefruit sections | 375 mL |
| 1 | apple (sliced) | 1 |
| 2 tablespoons | raisins | 30 mL |
| ½ cup | orange juice | 125 mL |
| | Lettuce leaves | |

Prick cranberries with sharp fork. Combine with remaining ingredients, except lettuce. Marinate 4 to 6 hours or overnight, drain. Serve on crisp lettuce leaves.

**YIELD:** 5 servings
**EXCHANGE 1 SERVING:** 1 fruit
**CALORIES 1 SERVING:** 40

# Cranberry Salad

| 1 pkg. (⅝ oz.) | lo-cal lemon gelatin | 1 pkg. (20 g) |
| 1 tablespoon | sugar replacement | 15 mL |
| 1 ½ cups | boiling water | 375 mL |
| 1 | orange | 1 |
| ½ cup | cranberries | 125 mL |
| ½ cup | celery (chopped) | 125 mL |
| ½ cup | apple (chopped) | 125 mL |

Dissolve gelatin and sugar replacement in boiling water. Cool to consistency of beaten egg whites. Grind orange (with peel) and cranberries; combine with celery and apple. Fold into gelatin mixture. Pour into mold or serving bowl. Chill until firm.

**YIELD:**                        8 servings
**EXCHANGE 1 SERVING:**  1 fruit
**CALORIES 1 SERVING:**   24

# Queen's Layered Gelatin

| | | |
|---|---|---|
| 1 pkg. (⅝ oz.) | lo-cal strawberry gelatin | 1 pkg. (20 g) |
| | Vegetable cooking spray | |
| 1 pkg. (⅝ oz.) | lo-cal lemon gelatin | 1 pkg. (20 g) |
| 3 ounces | cream cheese | 90 g |
| 1 cup | lo-cal whipped topping | |
| | (prepared) | 250 mL |
| 1 pkg. (⅝ oz.) | lo-cal orange gelatin | 1 pkg. (20 g) |
| ½ cup | unsweetened crushed | |
| | pineapple (drained) | 125 mL |
| ½ cup | carrot (grated) | 125 mL |
| | shredded lettuce | |

Prepare strawberry gelatin as directed on package. Pour into 2-quart (2-L) mold coated with vegetable cooking spray. Chill until firm. Prepare lemon gelatin as directed on package. Set until consistency of beaten egg whites. Whip cream cheese until light and fluffy. Fold into prepared whipped topping. Fold cream cheese topping into lemon gelatin. Pour over strawberry gelatin in mold. Chill until firm. Prepare orange gelatin as directed on package. Set until consistency of beaten egg whites. Fold in pineapple and carrot. Pour over lemon gelatin in mold. Chill until firm. Serve on bed of shredded lettuce.

**YIELD:**                        8 servings
**EXCHANGE 1 SERVING:**  ½ vegetable
                                     1 fat
**CALORIES 1 SERVING:**   57

# Blueberry Salad

| | | |
|---|---|---|
| 1 ½ cups | fresh or frozen blueberries | 375 mL |
| 2 teaspoons | sugar replacement | 10 mL |
| 1 envelope | unflavored gelatin | 1 envelope |
| 2 teaspoons | lemon juice | 10 mL |
| 1 cup | unsweetened crushed pineapple (drained) | 250 mL |
| 1 cup | lo-cal whipped topping (prepared) | 250 mL |

Place blueberries in saucepan. Sprinkle with sugar replacement. Allow to rest 30 minutes at room temperature; drain. Add enough boiling water to make 2 cups (500 mL). Sprinkle unflavored gelatin over surface. Stir to dissolve. Cook over low heat for 2 to 3 minutes. Allow to rest until cool. Add lemon juice. Remove 1/3 cup (90 mL) from blueberry mixture. Chill until set; reserve. Fold pineapple into remaining gelatin; chill until firm. Whip reserved gelatin until frothy. Fold in prepared whipped topping. Spread over blueberry gelatin. Chill until set.

**YIELD:** 4 servings
**EXCHANGE 1 SERVING:** ½ fruit
**CALORIES 1 SERVING:** 24

# Cabbage-Pineapple Salad

| | | |
|---|---|---|
| 3 cups | cabbage (shredded) | 750 mL |
| 1 pound can | unsweetened pineapple (diced) | 500-g can |
| 2 tablespoons | sugar replacement | 30 mL |
| dash | salt | dash |
| ½ cup | lo-cal whipped topping (prepared) | 125 mL |

Combine cabbage and pineapple with juice, sugar replacement and salt. Stir to dissolve sugar. Allow to rest at room temperature for 1½ to 2 hours. Drain thoroughly. Fold topping into cabbage mixture.

**YIELD:** 4 servings
**EXCHANGE 1 SERVING:** ½ fruit
**CALORIES 1 SERVING:** 28

*Note:* Lo-cal whipped topping can be made by mixing non-dairy whipped topping with water.

# Fruit Bowl

| ¼ cup | cantaloupe balls | 60 mL |
| ⅛ cup | honeydew balls | 30 mL |
| ½ cup | watermelon balls | 125 mL |
| ¼ cup | fresh, unsweetened pineapple chunks | 60 mL |
| | salt | |
| | lo-cal French dressing | |
| | lettuce | |

Sprinkle each fruit with salt and French dressing. Combine all ingredients, except lettuce. Refrigerate 1 to 2 hours. Serve on small bed of lettuce.

**YIELD:** 1 serving
**EXCHANGE:** 1 fruit
**CALORIES:** 40

# Fruit Salad

| | | |
|---|---|---|
| 16-ounce can | unsweetened apricot halves | 500-g can |
| 16-ounce can | unsweetened pineapple chunks | 500-g can |
| 2 teaspoons | lemon juice | 10 mL |
| 1 teaspoon | cornstarch | 5 mL |
| 2 teaspoons | sugar replacement | 10 mL |
| 1 teaspoon | margarine | 5 mL |
| 1 | apple (chopped) | 1 |
| 1 | banana (sliced) | 1 |
| | lo-cal whipped topping | |

Drain juice from apricots and pineapple into saucepan; add lemon juice and cornstarch. Cook over low heat to thicken. Remove from heat; add sugar replacement and margarine. Stir to blend; cool slightly. Combine all fruit in bowl. Pour sauce over fruit.

**YIELD:** 6 servings
**EXCHANGE 1 SERVING:** 1 fruit
**CALORIES 1 SERVING:** 53
*Added Touch:* Top each serving with a dab of whipped topping.

# SAUCES AND SALAD DRESSINGS

## Tomato Sauce

firm red tomatoes (or canned tomatoes without seasonings)

Quarter the tomatoes. Place in large kettle. Push down with hands or back of spoon to render some juice. Bake at 325° F (165° C) until soft pulp remains. Spoon into blender. Blend until smooth. Seal in sterilized jars or freeze.

## Creole Sauce

| | | |
|---|---|---|
| 28-ounce can | tomato | 800-g can |
| 1 medium | onion (chopped) | 1 medium |
| 1 | green pepper | 1 |
| 1 teaspoon | paprika | 5 mL |
| ¼ teaspoon | marjoram | 2 mL |
| | salt and pepper to taste | |

Combine all ingredients and cook over low heat for 25 minutes.

**YIELD:**     2 cups (500 mL)
**EXCHANGE:**  1 vegetable
**CALORIES:**  25

# Italian Tomato Sauce

| | | |
|---|---|---|
| 6 | tomatoes (peeled and cubed) | 6 |
| ¼ cup | green pepper (chopped) | 60 mL |
| ¼ cup | onion (chopped) | 60 mL |
| 2 T. | parsley (chopped) | 30 mL |
| 1 T. | lemon juice | 15 mL |
| dash each | oregano, marjoram, thyme, crushed bay leaf, horseradish | dash each |
| | salt and pepper to taste | |

Combine all ingredients in blender. Whip until smooth. Add enough water to make 2 cups (500 mL).

**YIELD:** 2 cups (500 mL)
**EXCHANGE:** 2 vegetables
**CALORIES:** 10

# Chili Sauce

| | | |
|---|---|---|
| 28-ounce can | tomatoes | 800-g can |
| 1 medium | apple | 1 medium |
| 1 medium | onion | 1 medium |
| 1 small | green pepper | 1 small |
| 1 cup | wine vinegar | 250 mL |
| ½ cup | sugar replacement | 125 mL |
| 1 tablespoon | salt | 15 mL |
| ½ teaspoon | ground clove | 3 mL |
| ½ teaspoon | cinnamon | 3 mL |
| ½ teaspoon | nutmeg | 3 mL |

Mash tomatoes; pour into kettle. Grind together apple, onion, green pepper, and vinegar. Add to kettle; cook until thick. Remove from heat. Add sugar replacement and seasonings. Return to heat; cook 5 minutes, stirring constantly.

**YIELD:** 2 cups (500 mL)
**EXCHANGE ½ CUP (125 ML):** 1 fruit
**CALORIES ½ CUP (125 ML):** 45

## VARIATIONS FOR ITALIAN DRESSING

To ½ cup (125 mL) lo-cal Italian dressing, add:

*Anchovy*
Mash 1 ounce (30 g) anchovy fillets. *Exchange:* 1 meat

*Bacon*
Grind 1 tablespoon (15 mL) Bacos; allow to mellow several hours.
*Exchange:* ½ fat

*Parmesan*
Add 1 tablespoon (15 mL) Parmesan cheese; allow to mellow several hours
*Exchange:* 1/8 meat

*Tomato*
Add 1 tablespoon (15 mL) tomato purée.

*Wine*
Add 1 tablespoon (15 mL) dry white or red wine.

**Calories ½ cup (125mL):** 24

## VARIATIONS FOR FRENCH DRESSING

To ½ cup (125 mL) lo-cal French dressing, add:

*Avocado*
Mash avocado to make 2 tablespoons (30 mL) *Exchange:* 1 fat

*Cheese*
Mash bleu cheese or Roquefort cheese to make 2 tablespoons (30 mL)
*Exchange:* ¼ meat

*Egg*
Crumble 1 hard-cooked egg yolk; combine with dash of hot pepper sauce
*Exchange:* 1 meat

*Lemon*
Add 1 tablespoon (15 mL) lemon juice.

*Soy Sauce*
Add 1 tablespoon (15 mL) soy sauce.

**Calories ½ cup (125 mL):** 100

## VARIATIONS FOR BLEU CHEESE DRESSING

To ½ cup (125 mL) lo-cal bleu cheese dressing, add:

*Anchovy*
Mash 1 ounce (30 g) anchovy fillets *Exchange:* 1 meat

*Bacon*
Grind 1 tablespoon (15 mL) Bacos; allow to mellow several hours.
*Exchange* ½ fat

*Chive*
Chop chives to make 2 tablespoons (30 mL); allow to mellow several hours.

*Herb*
Combine 1 teaspoon (5 mL) each ground parsley, chives, and marjoram.

**Calories ½ cup (125 mL):** 56

# Salad Dressing

| | | |
|---|---|---|
| 1½ cups | cold water | 375 mL |
| ¼ cup | vinegar | 60 mL |
| 1½ teaspoons | salt | 7 mL |
| 1 teaspoon | yellow mustard | 5 mL |
| 2 tablespoons | flour | 30 mL |
| 1 | egg (well beaten) | 1 |
| ¼ cup | sugar replacement | 60 mL |
| 2 teaspoons | margarine | 10 mL |

Combine cold water, vinegar, salt, mustard, flour, and egg in top of double boiler. Stir to blend. Cook until thick. Remove from heat. Add sugar replacement and margarine. Stir to blend.

**YIELD:** 1 cup (250 ml)
**EXCHANGE 2 TABLESPOONS (30 mL):** ½ vegetable
½ fat
**CALORIES 2 TABLESPOONS (30 mL):** 31

# Sweet Yogurt Dressing

| | | |
|---|---|---|
| 1 cup | lo-cal yogurt | 250 mL |
| ½ teaspoon | mace | 2 mL |
| 2 teaspoons | sugar replacement | 10 mL |
| dash | salt | dash |
| ½ cup | lo-cal whipped topping (prepared) | 125 mL |

Drain yogurt; beat until smooth and fluffy. Add mace, sugar replacement, and salt. Beat until blended. Fold in prepared whipped topping. Place in refrigerator until ready to serve. Good on fruit or gelatin salads.

**YIELD:** 1 cup (250 mL)
**EXCHANGE:** 1 milk
**CALORIES:** 100

# Herb Yogurt Dressing

| | | |
|---|---|---|
| 1 cup | lo-cal yogurt | 250 mL |
| 2 tablespoons | vinegar | 30 mL |
| 1 teaspoon | onion (grated) | 5 mL |
| 1 teaspoon | celery seeds | 5 mL |
| 1 teaspoon | dry mustard | 5 mL |
| 1 teaspoon | salt | 5 mL |
| ½ teaspoon | thyme | 2 mL |
| | salt and pepper to taste | |

Beat yogurt until smooth. Add remaining ingredients; blend well. Cover. Allow to rest at least 1 hour before serving.

**YIELD:** 1 cup (250 mL)
**EXCHANGE:** 1 milk
**CALORIES:** 86

# Bay Salad Dressing

| | | |
|---|---|---|
| 3 T. | liquid shortening | 45 mL |
| ½ cup | onion (finely chopped) | 125 mL |
| 2 T. | fresh parsley (finely chopped) | 30 mL |
| 2 T. | celery with leaves (finely chopped) | 30 mL |
| 1 | bay leaf | 1 |
| dash each | thyme, mace, rosemary | dash each |
| 2 T. | white wine | 30 mL |
| 1 cup | yogurt | 250 mL |
| 2 T. | skim milk | 30 mL |
| | salt and pepper to taste | |

Heat liquid shortening in small skillet. Add onion, parsley, celery, and seasonings. Cook over very low heat, stirring constantly, for 15 minutes. DO NOT ALLOW VEGETABLES TO BURN. Set aside to cool. Add wine; stir to mix. Allow to rest 30 minutes. strain, reserving liquid. Beat yogurt with skim milk.  Continue beating, adding wine liquid. Add salt and pepper. Blend.

**YIELD:** 1½ cups (375 mL)
**EXCHANGE ¼ CUP (60 mL):** ½ vegetable
½ fat
**CALORIES ¼ CUP (60 mL):** 44

# Tangy Barbecue Sauce

| | | |
|---|---|---|
| 1 cup | Chili Sauce (p. 144) | 250 mL |
| 2 tablespoons | lemon juice | 30 mL |
| 1 tablespoon | Worcestershire sauce | 15 mL |
| 1 teaspoon | horseradish | 5 mL |
| 1 teaspoon | Dijon mustard | 5 mL |
| 1 tablespoon | brown sugar replacement | 15 mL |
| dash each | hot pepper sauce, soy sauce, salt, pepper | dash each |

Combine all ingredients; stir to blend well.

**YIELD:** 1 cup (250 mL)
**EXCHANGE:** 2 fruit
**CALORIES:** 90

# Hollandaise Sauce

| | | |
|---|---|---|
| 1 | egg yolk | 1 |
| 1 tablespoon | evaporated (regular or skim) milk | 15 mL |
| 1/8 teaspoon | salt | 1 mL |
| dash | cayenne pepper | dash |
| 1 tablespoon | lemon juice | 15 mL |
| 1 tablespoon | margarine | 15 mL |

In the top of a double boiler, heat egg yolk, evaporated milk, salt, and cayenne pepper until thick. Place over hot water. Beat lemon juice into egg mixture until thick and creamy. Remove double boiler from heat. Add margarine, 1 teaspoon (5 mL) at a time. Beat until margarine is melted and blended in.

**YIELD:** ½ cup (125 mL)
**EXCHANGE:** ½ high-fat meat
3 fat
**CALORIES:** 213

# White Sauce

| | | |
|---|---|---|
| 2 tablespoons | margarine | 30 mL |
| 1½ tablespoons | flour | 25 mL |
| ¼ teaspoon | salt | 1 mL |
| 1 teaspoon | Worcestershire sauce | 5 mL |
| 1 cup | skim milk | 250 mL |

Melt margarine. Add flour, salt, and Worcestershire sauce. Blend thoroughly. Add skim milk. Cook until slightly thickened.

**YIELD:** 1 cup (250 mL)
**EXCHANGE ½ CUP (125 ML):** 1 bread
½ high-fat meat
**CALORIES ½ CUP (125 ML):** 190

# Orange Sauce

| | | |
|---|---|---|
| ½ teaspoon | cornstarch | 2 mL |
| 2 tablespoons | cold water | 30 mL |
| ½ cup | orange juice concentrate | 125 mL |
| 2 teaspoons | unsweetened orange drink mix | 10 mL |

Dissolve cornstarch in cold water. Add orange juice concentrate and drink mix. Cook over low heat until slightly thickened. Use as glaze on poultry or pork.

**YIELD:** ½ cup (125 mL)
**EXCHANGE:** 1 fruit
**CALORIES:** 52

# Teriyaki Marinade

| ⅓ cup | soy sauce | 80 mL |
| 2 tablespoons | wine vinegar | 30 mL |
| 2 tablespoons | sugar replacement | 30 mL |
| 2 teaspoons | salt | 10 mL |
| 1 teaspoon | ginger (powdered) | 5 mL |
| ½ teaspoon | garlic powder | 2 mL |

Blend well. No calories.

# SANDWICH SPREADS AND SNACKS

## Beef Tongue Spread

| | | |
|---|---|---|
| 6 ounces | cooked beef tongue (chopped) | 180 g |
| 2 tablespoons | Chili Sauce (p. 144) | 30 mL |
| 1 tablespoon | onion (finely chopped) | 15 mL |

Combine all ingredients; blend well.

**YIELD:** 1 cup (250 mL)
**EXCHANGE ¼ CUP (60 ML):** 1 medium-fat meat
**CALORIES ¼ CUP (60 ML):** 76

## Sweet Spread

| | | |
|---|---|---|
| ½ cup | margarine | 125 mL |
| 1 teaspoon | cinnamon | 5 mL |
| 1 teaspoon | orange rind (grated) | 5 mL |
| ½ teaspoon | nutmeg | 2 mL |
| 2 tablespoons | sugar replacement | 30 mL |

Have margarine at room temperature. Beat until light and fluffy. Add remaining ingredients. Beat until blended.

**YIELD:** 24 servings
**EXCHANGE 1 TEASPOON (5 ML):** 1 fat
**CALORIES 1 TEASPOON (5 ML):** 45

# Waldorf Sandwich Spread

| | | |
|---|---|---|
| ¼ cup | celery (finely chopped) | 60 mL |
| 1 small | apple (finely chopped) | 1 small |
| 1 T. | raisins (finely chopped) | 15 mL |
| 6 | walnut halves (finely chopped) | 6 |
| 2 T. | Salad Dressing (p. 146) | 30 mL |
| | salt to taste | |

Combine all ingredients; blend well.

**YIELD:** ½ cup (125 mL)
**EXCHANGE ¼ CUP (60 mL):** 1 fruit
1 fat
**CALORIES ¼ CUP (60 mL):** 96

# Tacos

| | | |
|---|---|---|
| 3 ounces | lean ground beef | 90 g |
| | salt and pepper to taste | |
| 1 tablespoon | taco sauce | 15 mL |
| 3 | 6-inch (15-cm) taco shells | 3 |
| 1½ ounces | Cheddar cheese (grated) 45 g | |
| 1½ tablespoons | onion (chopped) | 25 mL |
| 1 medium | tomato (chopped) | 1 medium |
| 1 cup | lettuce (shredded) | 250 mL |

Brown beef over low heat. Add salt and pepper. Drain. Add taco sauce; mix well. Divide beef mixture evenly among warm crisp shells. Top with cheese, onion, tomato, and lettuce.

**YIELD:** 1 serving
**EXCHANGE:** 1 bread
4 ½ meat
1 vegetable
**CALORIES 1 TACO:** 145

# Tuna Spread

| | | |
|---|---|---|
| 6½-ounce can | tuna (in water) | 200-mL can |
| 2 tablespoons | onion (finely chopped) | 30 mL |
| 2 tablespoons | celery (finely chopped) | 30 mL |
| 1 tablespoon | carrot (finely chopped) | 15 mL |
| ¼ cup | lo-cal bleu cheese dressing | 60 mL |
| | salt and pepper to taste | |

Drain tuna; chop fine. Add remaining ingredients and mix well.

**YIELD:**  1 cup (250 mL)
**EXCHANGE ¼ CUP (60 mL):**  1 lean meat
**CALORIES ¼ CUP (60 mL):**  48

# Blueberry Preserves
### (Strawberry-Raspberry)

| | | |
|---|---|---|
| 1 cup | fresh or frozen blueberries (unsweetened) | 250 mL |
| 1 teaspoon | lo-cal pectin | 5 mL |
| 1 teaspoon | sugar replacement | 5 mL |

Place blueberries in top of double boiler. Cook over boiling water until soft and juicy. (Crush berries against sides of double boiler.) Add pectin and sugar replacement. Blend in thoroughly. Cook until medium thick. Preserves can also be made with strawberries or raspberries.

**MICROWAVE:** Place blueberries in glass bowl. Cook on High for 4 minutes until soft and juicy. (Crush berries against sides of bowl.) Add pectin and sugar. Blend in thoroughly. Cook on High 30 seconds.

**YIELD:**  ⅔ cup (180 mL)
**EXCHANGE:** 1 fruit
**CALORIES:** 40

# Hamburger Relish

| | | |
|---|---|---|
| 2 quarts | cucumbers (ground) | 2 L |
| 2 | onions | 2 |
| 2 | green peppers | 2 |
| 1 | red pepper | 1 |
| ¼ cup | salt | 60 mL |
| 2 cups | vinegar | 500 mL |
| 1 teaspoon | mustard seeds | 5 mL |
| 1 teaspoon | celery seeds | 5 mL |
| 1 teaspoon | parsley flakes | 5 mL |
| 1 teaspoon | turmeric | 5 mL |
| 2 cups | sugar replacement | 500 mL |

Grind cucumbers, onions, green peppers, and red pepper. Stir in salt. Soak overnight; drain. Combine vinegar, mustard seeds, celery seeds, parsley flakes, and turmeric. Bring to a boil; cook for 10 minutes. Add ground vegetables; cook for 20 minutes. Remove from heat. Add sugar replacement; stir to dissolve. Allow to rest 24 hours; stir often. Drain slightly if too much liquid accumulates. Pack in scalded jars; seal.

**YIELD:** About 5 pints
**EXCHANGE 1 TABLESPOON (15 mL):** Negligible
**CALORIES 1 TABLESPOON (15 mL):** Negligible

# Beef Jerky

| 2 pounds | flank steak | 1 kg |
| ½ cup | soy sauce | 125 mL |
| | lemon pepper to taste | |
| | garlic salt to taste | |

Thoroughly chill flank steak. Cut into ¼ x 8-inch (6 x 20-cm) strips.  Combine soy sauce, lemon pepper, and garlic salt. Marinate steak in sauce for 24 hours; drain. Place on broiler pan. Bake at 150° F (66° C) for 10 to 12 hours, or until dry.

**EXCHANGE 2 STRIPS:**     1 high-fat meat
**CALORIES 2 STRIPS:**     108

# Teeny Pizza

| | dough for 1 biscuit | |
| 1 tablespoon | Tomato Sauce (p.143) | 30 mL |
| dash each | garlic powder, oregano, thyme, salt | dash each |
| ½ ounce | meat of your choice | 15 g |
| ½ ounce | mozzarella cheese (shredded) | 15 g |

Press or roll biscuit dough flat. Roll edge up or place in individual baking dish. Combine Tomato Sauce and seasonings. Spread over entire surface of biscuit.  Top with meat and cheese.  Bake at 450° F (230° C) for 10 minutes.

**YIELD:**       1 serving
**EXCHANGE:**  1 meat
                     1 bread
**CALORIES:**   150

# Wrapped Wiener

| | | |
|---|---|---|
| 1 | wiener | 1 |
| ³⁄₈-inch strip | cheese | 1-cm strip |
| | dough for 1 biscuit | |

Make a thin slit in wiener; insert strip of cheese in slit. Roll or pat biscuit dough thin. Place wiener on edge of dough; roll up. Secure by pinching dough together, or use a toothpick. Bake at 375° F (190° C) for 15 minutes, or until golden brown.

**YIELD:**   1 serving
**EXCHANGE**   1¼ meat
   1 bread
**CALORIES:**   141

# Fish Bundles

| | | |
|---|---|---|
| ½ cup | Herb-Seasoned Stuffing (p. 107) | 125 mL |
| 8 ounces | Cooked Flaked Fish (p. 80) | 240 g |
| 1 | egg | 1 |

Moisten stuffing with water. Allow to stand 5 minutes, or until soft. (Add extra water if needed.) Blend fish and egg into softened stuffing. Form into 6 patties. Broil for 10 to 15 minutes. Turn once.

**YIELD:**   6 patties
**EXCHANGE 1 PATTY:**   1 ¼ meat
   ¼ bread
   1/8 fat
**CALORIES 1 PATTY:**   45

# Garlic Dill Pickles

| | | |
|---|---|---|
| 3 cups | water | 750 mL |
| 3 cups | vinegar | 750 mL |
| ½ cup | pickling salt | 125 mL |
| | firm medium cucumbers (quartered) | |
| 1 per jar | dill head | 1 per jar |
| 1 per jar | garlic clove | 1 per jar |

Combine water, vinegar, and pickling salt. Bring to a boil; cook for 5 minutes. Divide cucumbers, dill, and garlic among three scalded 1 quart (1 L) jars. Fill jars with vinegar mixture. Seal immediately. Ready in 6 to 8 weeks.

**EXCHANGE 1 PICKLE:** Negligible
**CALORIES 1 PICKLE:** Negligible


# Bread and Butter Pickles

| | | |
|---|---|---|
| 4 quarts | cucumbers (sliced) | 4 L |
| 5 | onions | 5 |
| 1 quart | crushed ice | 1 L |
| ⅓ cup salt | 90 mL | |
| 2 cups | vinegar | 500 mL |
| 1½ teaspoons | turmeric | 7 mL |
| 1½ teaspoons | celery seeds | 7 mL |
| 2 teaspoons | mustard seeds | 10 mL |
| 1 teaspoon | ginger | 5 mL |
| 1½ cups | sugar replacement | 375 mL |

Slice cucumbers and onions; place in large saucepan. Mix ice and salt; stir into cucumbers and onions. Cover. Chill for 5 to 6 hours. Drain; remove ice. Combine vinegar and seasonings. Bring to a boil; simmer for 5 minutes. Add sugar replacement; stir to dissolve. Add drained cucumbers and onions. Bring to a boil. Put into scaled jars and seal.

# Dill Midgets

| | | |
|---|---|---|
| 1 head | dill | 1 head |
| 20 to 25 | firm midget cucumbers | 20 to 25 |
| ½ teaspoon | alum | 2 mL |
| 2 teaspoons | pickling salt | 10 mL |
| ½ cup | white vinegar | 125 mL |

Scald 1 pint (½ L) jar. Push dill head to bottom of jar. Fill with midgets. Add alum and pickling salt. Pour vinegar over top. Add enough cold water to fill jar; seal. Shake vigorously. Ready in 8 to 10 weeks.

**YIELD:** 20 to 25 pickles
**EXCHANGE 1 PICKLE:** Negligible
**CALORIES 1 PICKLE:** Negligible

# Russian Teasicles

| | | |
|---|---|---|
| 2 quarts | water | 2 L |
| 1 | cinnamon stick | 1 |
| 3 | whole cloves | 3 |
| 2 tablespoons | black tea leaves | 30 mL |
| 6-ounce can | frozen lemon juice (unsweetened) | 180-mL can |
| 6-ounce can | rozen orange juice | 180-mL can |
| ½ cup | sugar replacement | 125 mL |

Combine water, cinnamon stick, whole cloves, and black tea leaves in large kettle. Bring to a boil; reduce heat and simmer for 15 to 20 minutes. Strain; cool slightly. Add frozen concentrates and sugar replacement. Stir to dissolve. Pour into freezer stick trays; freeze.

**YIELD:** about 38 popsicles
**EXCHANGE 1 POPSICLE:** ½ fruit
**CALORIES 1 POPSICLE:** 5

# Egg Nog

| | | |
|---|---|---|
| 1 | egg (well beaten) | 1 |
| 2 teaspoons | sugar replacement | 30 mL |
| dash | salt, vanilla extract | dash |
| ¾ cup | cold milk | 180 mL |
| dash | nutmeg to taste | dash |

Combine egg with sugar replacement and salt. Add vanilla extract and cold milk. Beat well. Pour into glass or mug; sprinkle with nutmeg.

**YIELD:** 1 serving
**EXCHANGE:** 1 meat
1 milk
**CALORIES:** 148

# Special
# DESSERT
# Section

# CAKES, TORTS AND CAKE ROLLS

## Strawberry Topping
### (Blueberry-Raspberry)

| 2 cups | fresh or frozen strawberries (unsweetened) | 500 mL |
| 1½ teaspoons | cornstarch | 7 mL |
| ¼ cup | cold water | 60 mL |
| 2 teaspoons | sugar replacement | 10 mL |

Place strawberries in top of double boiler. Cook over boiling water until soft and juicy. Blend cornstarch and cold water. Add to strawberries. Cook until clear and slightly thickened. Remove from heat; add sugar replacement. Cool. Topping can also be made with blueberries or raspberries.

**YIELD:** 1 ½ cups (375 mL)
**EXCHANGE ½ CUP (125 mL):** 1 fruit
**CALORIES ½ CUP (125 mL):** 40

# Strawberry Shortcake

|  | dough for 1 biscuit |  |
|---|---|---|
| ½ cup | Strawberry Topping (p. 161) | 125 mL |
| ¼ cup | fresh strawberries (halved) | 60 mL |
| 2 tablespoons | lo-cal whipped topping (prepared) | 30 mL |

Bake biscuit as directed on package. Cool. Cut in half. Layer biscuit, half of the Strawberry Topping, and half of the strawberries; repeat. Top with prepared whipped topping.

**YIELD:** 1 serving
**EXCHANGE:** 1 bread
          1 ½ fruit
**CALORIES:** 100

# Banana Cake Roll

| 4 | eggs (separated) | 4 |
|---|---|---|
| 10 tablespoons | granulated sugar replacement | 150 mL |
| ½ teaspoon | vanilla extract | 2 mL |
| ⅔ cup cake flour (sifted)     180 mL | | |
| 1 teaspoon | baking powder | 5 mL |
| ¼ teaspoon | salt | 1 mL |
|  | Vegetable cooking spray |  |
| 1 package | loc-cal banana pudding (prepared) 1 package | |
|  | Chocolate Drizzle (p. 163) | |

Beat egg yolks until thick and lemon colored; gradually beat in 3 tablespoons (45 mL) of the sugar replacement. Add vanilla extract. Beat egg whites to soft peaks; gradually beat in the remaining sugar replacement; beat until stiff peaks form. Fold yolks into whites. Sift together cake flour, baking powder, and salt. Fold into egg mixture. Spread batter into

15½ x 10½ x 1-inch (39 x 25 x 3-cm) jelly-roll pan (coated with vegetable cooking spray and lightly floured). Bake at 375° F (190° C) for 10 to 15 minutes, or until done. Loosen sides and turn out on towel lightly sprinkled with a mixture of flour and sugar replacement. Roll up cake and towel from narrow end. Cool completely; unroll. Spread evenly with prepared banana pudding. Roll up. Frost with Chocolate Drizzle.

**YIELD:** 10 servings
**EXCHANGE 1 SERVING:** 1 bread
½ fruit
¼ milk
**CALORIES 1 SERVING:** 62

# Chocolate Drizzle

| | | |
|---|---|---|
| 2 teaspoons | cornstarch | 10 mL |
| ¼ cup | cold water | 60 mL |
| dash | salt | dash |
| 1 ounce | unsweetened chocolate | 30 g |
| ⅓ cup sugar replacement | | 90 mL |
| ½ teaspoon | butter | 3 mL |

Blend cornstarch and cold water. Pour into small saucepan. Add salt and chocolate. Cook on low heat until chocolate melts and mixture is thick. Remove from heat. Stir in sugar replacement. Blend in butter.

**YIELD:** ⅓ cup (90 mL)
**EXCHANGE:** Negligible
**CALORIES:** Negligible

# Rich Chocolate Cake

| | | |
|---|---|---|
| 1⅓ cups | cake flour | 340 mL |
| ⅓ cup | unsweetened cocoa powder | 90 mL |
| ¼ teaspoon | baking powder | 1 mL |
| ¼ teaspoon | baking soda | 1 mL |
| Pinch | salt (optional) | pinch |
| ½ cup | egg substitute | 125 mL |
| 1 teaspoon | vanilla extract | 5mL |
| 1 tablespoon | raspberry liqueur | 45 mL |
| ½ cup | nonfat buttermilk | 125 mL |
| 4 tablespoons | margarine or butter | 90 mL |
| 2 tablespoons | prune purée | 30 mL |
| 15 packets | concentrated acesulfame-K | 15 packets |
| 3 tablespoons | sugar | 45 mL |
| 6 | egg whites | 6 |
| ¼ teaspoon | cream of tartar | 1 mL |
| ½ cup | frozen raspberries | 125 mL |
| ½ teaspoon | concentrated aspartame | 2 mL |

Sift the first five ingredients together twice; set aside. Combine the egg substitute and vanilla extract, raspberry liqueur, and buttermilk. Using an electric mixer, cream the margarine or butter and the prune purée. Add acesulfame-K and sugar and beat well. Gradually add the egg substitute alternately with the flour mixture. Beat until well combined. Beat the egg whites until stiff. Add the cream of tartar and continue beating. Add a small amount of egg whites to the batter to lighten it. With a rubber spatula, fold in the remaining beaten whites. Pour into two 8-inch (20 cm) round cake pans that have been coated with non-stick cooking spray. Bake in a preheated 350° F (180° C) oven for 30 to 35 minutes. Cool, then invert onto a plate. Combine the raspberries and aspartame in a food processor to make raspberry purée. Spread raspberry puree over the top of one layer. Put the other layer on top and cover with raspberry purée. Decorate top with whole raspberries if desired.

**Yield:** 10 servings
**Exchanges:** 2 bread
½ fat
**Calories:** 189

# Angel Food Cake

| | | |
|---|---|---|
| 1 cup | flour | 250 mL |
| ¼ cup | sugar | 60 mL |
| 3 packets | concentrated acesulfame-K | 3 packets |
| 1½ cups | egg whites (12) | 375 mL |
| 1½ teaspoons | cream of tartar | 7 mL |
| ¼ teaspoon | salt | 60 mL |
| ¼ cup | sugar | 60 mL |
| 4 packets | concentrated acesulfame-K | 4 packets |
| 1½ teaspoons | vanilla extract | 7 mL |
| ½ teaspoon | almond extract | 2 mL |

Sift together the flour, ¼ cup of sugar, and 3 packets of ace-sulfame-K. Set aside. In a large mixing bowl, combine the egg whites, cream of tartar, and salt. With an electric mixer, beat until foamy. Mix together ¼ cup of sugar and 4 packets of the second acesulfame-K. Gradually add this mixture, a tablespoon (15 mL) at a time, to the egg whites. Continue beating until stiff peaks form. Fold in the vanilla and almond extracts. Sprinkle the flour mixture over the beaten egg whites. Fold gently just until the flour disappears. Fold the batter into an ungreased 10 x 4-inch (25 x 10-cm) tube pan.

Bake in a 375° F (190° C) oven for 30 to 35 minutes, until no imprint remains after finger lightly touches the top of the cake. The top should be golden brown. To cool, turn the baked cake over. For best results, stand the tube pan on a custard cup or put a bottle in the center hole to hold the top away from the counter so circulation will occur. Remove the cake from the pan only after it is thoroughly cool. Drizzle with bittersweet topping, fruit topping, or sliced fresh fruit.

**YIELD:**    24 slices
**EXCHANGE:**  ½ bread
**CALORIES:**  42
Plus calories and exchanges for topping

# Chocolate Éclair Cake

### Dough

| 1 cup | water | 250 mL |
|---|---|---|
| ½ cup | canola oil | 125 mL |
| 1 cup | flour | 250 mL |
| 4 | eggs | 4 |
| 1 teaspoon | butter-flavored extract | 5 mL |

### Filling

| 2 8-ounce | sugar-free vanilla pudding | 2 244-g packages |
|---|---|---|
| 2 ½ cups | skim milk | 625 mL |
| ¾ cup | prepared sugar-free, low-fat whipped topping from mix | 190 mL |

### Topping

| 6 tablespoons | unsweetened cocoa powder | 90 mL |
|---|---|---|
| 2 tablespoons | canola oil | 30 mL |
| 2 tablespoons | skim milk | 30 mL |
| ¾ cup | aspartame | 190 mL |
| 1 teaspoon | vanilla extract | 5 mL |
| | extra milk, if needed | |
| 1 teaspoon | butter-flavored extract | 5 mL |

**To make the dough:** Heat the water and oil to a rolling boil. Stir in the flour over low heat until the mixture forms a ball.

Remove from the heat. Using an electric mixer, beat in the eggs thoroughly, one at a time. Put in the butter extract. Spoon onto an ungreased cookie sheet in the shape of a ring or wreath. Bake until golden brown and dry at 400° F (200° C) for 35 to 40 minutes. Cool away from drafts. Slice in half horizontally. Just before serving add the filling by removing the top half, adding the filling, and replacing the top. Add the topping.

**To make the filling:** Whisk the pudding and milk until the mixture thickens. Fold in the whipped topping.

**To make the topping:** Melt the cocoa powder with the oil and milk. Cool. Add the aspartame and vanilla and beat until the mixture is the desired consistency. Add a little extra milk if necessary, one teaspoon at a time. Drizzle on top of the cake.

| YIELD: | 24 servings |
|---|---|
| EXCHANGE | 1 bread |
| | 1 fat |
| CALORIES: | 100 |

# Banana Tea Bread

| ½ cup | egg substitute | 125 mL |
|---|---|---|
| 1 cup | ripe banana, mashed | 250 mL |
| 1 teaspoon | vanilla extract | 5 mL |
| 2 cups | flour | 500 mL |
| ½ teaspoon | salt | 2 mL |
| 1 teaspoon | baking soda | 5 mL |
| 2 tablespoons | sugar | 30 mL |
| 6 packets | concentrated acesulfame-K | 6 packets |

## Glaze

| | | |
|---|---|---|
| 2 tablespoons | boiling water | 30 mL |
| 4 teaspoons | concentrated aspartame | 20 mL |

Beat the egg substitute with a wire whisk; add the mashed banana and vanilla extract. Sift together the flour, salt, baking soda, sugar, and acesulfame-K. Add these dry ingredients to the egg-banana mixture and stir. Turn the mixture into a loaf pan that has been coated with non-stick cooking spray. Bake in a preheated 350° F (180° C) oven for 40 minutes.

After the bread is out of the oven, poke holes all over the top using a fork. Combine boiling water and aspartame; and use a pastry brush to cover top with glaze, letting the glace sink into the holes.

**YIELD:** 20 servings
**EXCHANGE:** 1 bread
**CALORIES:** 66

# Mocha Chocolate Roll

| | | |
|---|---|---|
| 1 cup | sifted cake flour | 250 mL |
| ¼ cup | unsweetened cocoa powder | 60 mL |
| 1 teaspoon | baking powder | 5 mL |
| 3 | eggs | 3 |
| ¼ cup | sugar | 60 mL |
| 3 packets | concentrated acesulfame-K | 3 packets |
| ⅓ cup cold coffee | 90 mL | |
| 1 teaspoon | vanilla extract | 5mL |

## Filling

| | | |
|---|---|---|
| 1 package | sugar-free whipped topping mix | 1 package |
| ½ cup | cold, very strong coffee | 125 mL |

Spray a 15 x 10 x 1-inch (37 x 25 x 3-cm) jelly-roll pan; line the bottom with wax paper; spray the paper. Sift the flour, cocoa, and baking powder together. With an electric mixer, beat the eggs in a medium bowl until thick and creamy and light in color. Gradually add the sugar and acesulfame-K, beating constantly until the mixture is very thick. Stir in the coffee and vanilla extract. Fold in the flour mixture. Spread the batter evenly in a prepared pan.

Bake in a 350° F (180° C) oven for 12 minutes or until the center springs back when pressed lightly with a fingertip. Loosen the cake around the edges with a knife; invert the pan onto a clean tea towel. Peel off the wax paper. Starting at the short end, roll up the cake and towel together. Place the roll, seam-side down, on a wire rack; cool completely.

To make the filling, follow the directions for the whipped topping mix on the package but use cold coffee instead of water. When the cake is cool, unroll it carefully. Spread it evenly with filling. To start rerolling, lift the cake with the end of the towel. Place it, seam-side down, on a serving plate.

**YIELD:**      20 servings
**EXCHANGE:** ½ bread
               ½ fat
**CALORIES:**  70

# French Pastry Cake

| | | |
|---|---|---|
| ½ cup | margarine or butter | 125 mL |
| ½ cup | nonfat cream cheese | 125 mL |
| ¼ cup | sugar | 60 mL |
| ½ cup | measures-like-sugar saccharin | 125 mL |
| 2 | eggs or equivalent egg substitute | 2 |
| 1 cup | nonfat sour cream | 250 mL |
| 1 cup | nonfat mayonnaise | 250 mL |
| 1 tablespoon | vanilla extract | 15 mL |
| 2 cups | flour | 500 mL |
| 1 teaspoon | baking powder | 5 mL |
| 1 teaspoon | baking soda | 5 mL |

## Cinnamon Mixture

| | | |
|---|---|---|
| 1 tablespoon | cinnamon | 15 mL |
| 2 packets | concentrated acesulfame-K | 2 packets |
| ½ cup | chopped almonds | ½ cup |

Cream margarine or butter and cream cheese with sugar and saccharin. Add the eggs, sour cream, mayonnaise, and vanilla extract; beat well. Mix the flour, baking powder, and baking soda and add to the batter. Put half the batter into a tube pan or bundt pan coated with non-stick cooking spray. Mix together the cinnamon, acesulfame-K, and chopped almonds. Sprinkle half the cinnamon mixture on top of the batter in the pan, then add the rest of the batter. Sprinkle the rest of the cinnamon mixture on top of the batter. Bake at 350° F (180° C) 60 to 75 minutes or until the top is light brown and the cake pulls away from the pan.

**YIELD:** 20 servings
**EXCHANGE:** 1 fat
1 bread
**CALORIES:** 155

# CHEESECAKES

## Granola Cheesecake

### Crust

| | | |
|---|---|---|
| ¼ cup | margarine or butter, melted | 60 mL |
| 1 tablespoon | water | 15 mL |
| 3 packets | concentrated acesulfame-K | 3 packets |
| 1 cup | Granola Topping | 250 mL |

### Filling

| | | |
|---|---|---|
| 8 ounces | nonfat cream cheese, softened | 250 mL |
| 1 cup | nonfat cottage cheese, drained | 250 mL |
| ½ cup | egg substitute or 2 eggs | 125 mL |
| 3 packets | concentrated acesulfame-K | 3 packets |
| 1 teaspoon | vanilla extract | 5 mL |
| 1 tablespoon | flour | 15 mL |

### Topping

| | | |
|---|---|---|
| 1/3 cup | Granola Topping | 90 mL |

Stir the crust ingredients together and press the mixture into the bottom of a 9-inch (23-cm) springform pan. Set aside. Beat the filling ingredients together until smooth. Spoon this carefully over the crust. Sprinkle the top with granola topping. Bake in a 375° F (190° C) oven for 40 minutes or until set. Cool before removing cake from the pan.

YIELD:      10 servings
EXCHANGE:  1 meat
CALORIES:   88

# Healthy Cheesecake

| ¼ cup | graham cracker crumbs | 60 mL |
|---|---|---|
| 2 cups | yogurt cheese* | 500 mL |
| 2 teaspoons | vanilla extract | 10 mL |
| ½ cup | egg substitute | 125 mL |
| 2 tablespoons | cornstarch | 30 mL |
| 6 packets | concentrated acesulfame-K | 6 packets |

### Topping

| ½ cup | nonfat sour cream | 125 mL |
|---|---|---|
| 2 teaspoons | sugar | 10 mL |
| 2 teaspoons | concentrated acesulfame-K | 2 t |
| 1 teaspoon | vanilla extract | 5 mL |

Spray a 9-inch (23-cm) springform pan with non-stick cooking spray. Sprinkle it evenly with gram-cracker crumbs. Set aside.

Use an electric mixer to combine the next five ingredients. Beat until creamy. Pour the mixture onto the crumbs. Bake in a preheated 325° F (160° C) oven for 35 minutes. Remove from the oven and let cool. Refrigerate. Combine the topping ingredients and pour the mixture over the baked, chilled cheesecake. Return it to the oven for 10 minutes. Chill. Run a knife around the edge of the pan to loosen the cheesecake.

YIELD:      12 servings
EXCHANGE:  ½ bread
CALORIES:   49

* Yogurt cheese is made by letting yogurt drip through cheesecloth overnight in the refrigerator.

# Apple Cheesecake

| | | |
|---|---|---|
| 1 pound | nonfat cottage cheese | 450 g |
| 2/3 cup | nonfat sour cream | 180 mL |
| 4 t. | fructose | 20 mL |
| 2 | eggs | 2 |
| 1 T. | all-purpose flour | 15 mL |
| ½ t. | nutmeg | 5 mL |
| pinch | cinnamon | pinch |
| 1 | juice of one lemon | 1 |
| 4 | small apples, peeled, cored, and sliced into half moons | 4 |
| | Graham-Cracker Crust (page 190) | (optional) |

Spray a 9-inch (23-cm) springform pan with non-stick cooking spray. Sprinkle it evenly with gram-cracker crumbs. Set aside.

Beat the cottage cheese, sour cream, fructose, eggs, flour, nutmeg, and cinnamon until smooth. Stir in the lemon juice. Spread half the apples in the bottom, over a crust if you like. Pour the cottage cheese mixture over the apples. Top with the remaining apples. Bake in a preheated oven at 375° F (190° C) or until set. Cool completely.

**YIELD:** 10 servings
**EXCHANGE:** 1 bread
**CALORIES:** 101
Plus calories and exchanges for crust

# Cheesecake with Jelly Glaze

| | | |
|---|---|---|
| 1 8-oz. pkg. | nonfat cream cheese | 1 250-mL pkg. |
| 1 cup | nonfat yogurt sweetened with aspartame | 250 mL |
| 1 pkg. | unsweetened gelatin | 1 package |
| ¼ cup | water | 90 mL |
| 1 T. | measures-like-sugar aspartame | 15 mL |
| 1 cup | fresh fruit, or canned, no sugar added | 250 mL |
| 3 T. | jelly, made with saccharin | 45 mL |

Combine the cream cheese and yogurt and beat until smooth. In a small saucepan, sprinkle the gelatin into the water; let soften for 2 minutes. Over low heat, stir to dissolve the gelatin. Remove from the heat and add to cream cheese mixture. Add the aspartame. With an electric mixer, beat until smooth. Pour into a crust of your choice (A graham-cracker crust is traditional.) Arrange the fruit on top. Microwave the jelly for 30 seconds or heat in a saucepan over low heat. When jelly is liquefied, use a pastry brush to glaze the top of the cheesecake.

**YIELD:** 8 servings  **CALORIES:** 60
**EXCHANGE:** 1 milk
Plus calories and exchanges for crust

# Pumpkin Cheesecake

| | | |
|---|---|---|
| 1 pound | nonfat cream cheese | 450 g |
| 12 teaspoons | fructose | 60 mL |
| ¼ cup | egg substitute | 60 mL |
| 1 16-ounce can | pumpkin | 1 488-mL can |
| 1½ teaspoons | cinnamon | 7.5 mL |
| 1 teaspoon | allspice | 5 mL |
| ¼ teaspoon | ginger | 1.25 mL |
| ¼ teaspoon | mace | 1.25 mL |
| 1 | unbaked crust, preferably graham cracker | 1 |

Spray an 8-inch (20-cm) springform pan with nonstick veg-etable cooking spray. Line the bottom of the sprayed pan with crust, if desired. Beat the cream cheese, fructose, and egg substitute until smooth. Beat the pumpkin and spices into the cheese mixture. Spoon the filling into the crust, if used. Bake in a preheated 350° F (180° C) oven for 45 min-utes or until set. Cool the cake completely before removing it from the pan.

**YIELD:**      10 servings
**EXCHANGE:**  1 milk
**CALORIES:**   82
Plus calories and exchanges for crust

# Ricotta Pie

| | | |
|---|---|---|
| 2 pounds | fat-free ricotta | 900 g |
| 6 | eggs | 6 |
| ⅓ cup | sugar | 90 mL |
| ⅓ cup | measures-like-sugar saccharin | 90 mL |
| 2 teaspoons | vanilla extract | 10 mL |
| 2 teaspoons | butter-flavored extract | 10 mL |
| 1 teaspoon | cinnamon | 5 mL |

With an electric mixer, beat all the ingredients except the cinnamon until smooth. Pour the batter into a 10-inch (25-cm) pie crust of your choice. Sprinkle with cinnamon. Bake at 350° F (180° C) for 50 to 60 minutes until a knife insert-ed comes out clean. Cool. Refrigerate.

**YIELD:**      8 servings
**EXCHANGE:**  1 ½ milk
              1 meat
**CALORIES:**   159
Plus calories and exchanges for crust

# No-Bake Orange Cheesecake

## Crust

| | | |
|---|---|---|
| 1 cup | finely crushed graham cracker crumbs | 250 mL |
| 3 T. | melted margarine or butter | 45 mL |

## Cheesecake Filling

| | | |
|---|---|---|
| ¼ cup | cold water | 60 mL |
| 1 envelope | unflavored gelatin | 1 envelope |
| 16 ounces | nonfat cream cheese, at room temperature | 450 g |
| ¼ cup | sugar | 60 mL |
| 6 packets | concentrated acesulfame-K | 6 packets |
| 1 cup | nonfat sour cream | 250 mL |
| ¾ cup | freshly squeezed orange juice | 180 mL |
| 1 teaspoon | freshly grated orange peel | 5 mL |
| 2 teaspoons | orange flavoring | 10 mL |

## Topping

| | | |
|---|---|---|
| 3 | navel oranges, peeled, bitter parts removed | 3 |

**To make the crust:** Mix the graham-cracker crumbs and margarine. Spread this over the bottom and a little up the sides of a 9-inch (23-cm) springform pan. Freeze the crust while mixing the filling.

**To make the filling:** Put the water in a small saucepan and sprinkle the gelatin on top. After 1 minute, turn the heat on low and, stirring constantly, heat for 2-3 minutes until the gelatin is dissolved. Remove from heat.

With an electric mixer, beat the cream cheese, sugar, and acesulfame-K in a large bowl. When the mixture is fluffy, add the sour cream and beat well. Mix in the orange juice, gelatin, peel, and flavoring. Pour into a chilled crust. Refrigerate for 4 to 6 hours until firm.

Before serving, run a thin knife around the edge of the cake to loosen it. Remove the springform from the outside. Top the cake with sliced oranges.

**YIELD:** 12 servings
**EXCHANGE:** 1 bread
           ½ fat
           ½ milk
**CALORIES:** 164

# Creamy Amaretto Cheesecake

| | | |
|---|---|---|
| 2 8-oz. pkg. | nonfat cream cheese | 2 244-g pkg. |
| 2 tablespoons | cornstarch 30 mL | |
| 2 teaspoons | concentrated acesulfame-K | 10 mL |
| 2 tablespoons | sugar | 30 mL |
| ¼ cup | Amaretto | 60 mL |
| 1 teaspoon | vanilla extract | 5 mL |
| ½ cup | egg substitute | 125 mL |
| 1 | graham cracker crust (optional) | 1 |
| | fresh fruit (optional) | |

Cream the first six ingredients together. Pour in the egg substitute and beat with an electric mixer until creamy. Pour the batter into an 8-inch (20-cm) graham-cracker crust, or lightly coat an 8-inch pi plate with nonfat vegetable spray.. Bake in a preheated 325° F (160° C) oven for 35 minutes. Chill. Before serving, top with fruit, if desired.

**YIELD:** 8 servings
**EXCHANGE:** 1 milk
**CALORIES:** 108
Plus calories and exchanges for graham-cracker crust

# Strawberry Cream Cheese Tarts

| | | |
|---|---|---|
| 6 ounces | nonfat cream cheese | 200 g |
| ¾ cup | nonfat cottage cheese | 190 mL |
| ⅔ cup | nonfat sour cream | 180 mL |
| 3 | eggs separated | 3 |
| 7 teaspoons | fructose | 35 mL |
| 1 | graham cracker crust recipe | 1 |
| | Pressed into 18 mini tart pans | |

To prepare the filling, beat the cream cheese, cottage cheese, sour cream, egg yolks, and fructose in a large bowl until smooth. In another bowl, beat the egg whites until soft peaks form; fold them into the cheese mixture. Spoon the filling into the prepared crusts. Chill until set. Garnish with Strawberry Topping, (page 161).

**YIELD:** 18 tarts
**EXCHANGE:** ½ milk
**CALORIES:** 44

# Marble Cheesecake

| | | |
|---|---|---|
| 2 cups | nonfat ricotta cheese | 500 mL |
| 8 ounces | nonfat cream cheese | 250 g |
| ¼ cup | egg substitute | 60 mL |
| 3 | egg whites | 3 |
| 2 tablespoons | sugar | 30 mL |
| 12 packets | concentrated acesulfame-K | 12 packets |
| 1 tablespoon | vanilla extract | 15 mL |
| 1½ teaspoons | lemon juice | 7.5 mL |
| 3 tablespoons | cocoa | 45 mL |
| 3 tablespoons | water | 45 mL |
| 2 packets | concentrated acesulfame-K | 2 packets |
| 3 tablespoons | crumbs made from chocolate cookies sweetened with fructose | 45 mL |

Put the ricotta cheese in a food processor or blender and process for a full minute. Soften the cream cheese in a microwave oven for 30 seconds. Add it to the food processor with the egg substitute, egg whites, sugar, 12 packets of acesulfame-K, vanilla extract, and lemon juice. Process to combine. In a medium bowl, whisk together the cocoa, water, and 2 packets of acesulfame-K.

Pour approximately 1 cup (250 mL) cheese batter from the food processor into the cocoa. Whisk to combine. Set aside this "chocolate" batter. Then take a 9-inch (23-cm) springform baking pan that has been sprayed with nonstick vegetable cooking spray. Pour most of the white batter into this prepared pan. Pour all the chocolate batter in the center on top of the white batter. There will be a white ring all around the edge of the pan. Carefully pour the rest of the white batter into the center of the chocolate batter. Use a knife to marble the batters by making an "S" curve through the batter. Do not mix completely.

Place the springform pan in the center of a baking pan. Slowly and carefully pour boiling water into the outer baking pan, smoothing the batter in the springform pan. (This hot-water bath will help the cheesecake bake like a custard.) Bake in a preheated 325° F (160° C) oven for 50 minutes or until it starts to shrink away from the sides of the pan. Remove the cake from the hot-water bath and chill it completely overnight. Press chocolate cookie crumbs onto the sides of the cake.

**YIELD:**      16 servings
**EXCHANGE:** ½ milk
**CALORIES:**   57

# COOKIES, SQUARES, AND OTHER FINGER FOOD

## Oatmeal Cookies

| | | |
|---|---|---|
| 1 cup | flour | 250 mL |
| ½ teaspoon | salt | 2 mL |
| ½ teaspoon | baking powder | 2 mL |
| ¼ teaspoon | baking soda | 2 mL |
| ½ teaspoon | cinnamon | 3 mL |
| ½ teaspoon | nutmeg | 2 mL |
| ½ cup | raisins | 125 mL |
| 1½ cups | oatmeal | 375 mL |
| ½ cup | sugar replacement | 125 mL |
| ½ cup | margarine (melted) | 125 mL |
| 1 | egg | 1 |
| ½ cup | skim milk | 125 mL |

Combine flour, salt, baking powder, baking soda, cinnamon, nutmeg, raisins, and oatmeal. Mix thoroughly. Beat in sugar replacement, melted margarine, egg, and skim milk. (Add small amount of water if dough is too stiff.) Drop by teaspoonfuls onto cookie sheet. Bake at 400° F (200° C) for 10 minutes.

| | |
|---|---|
| **YIELD:** | 36 cookies |
| **EXCHANGE 1 COOKIE:** | ½ bread |
| | ¼ fat |
| **CALORIES 1 COOKIE:** | 37 |

# Cookie Cutter Cookies

| | | |
|---|---|---|
| 1 cup | margarine or butter | 350 mL |
| ¼ cup | sugar | 60 mL |
| 6 packets | concentrated acesulfame-K | 6 packets |
| 2½ cups | flour | 625 mL |
| 1 teaspoon | baking soda | 5 mL |
| 1 teaspoon | cream of tartar | 5 mL |
| 1 teaspoon | vanilla extract | 5 mL |
| 1 teaspoon | almond extract | 5 mL |
| 1 | egg or equivalent egg substitute | 1 |

Cream the margarine and sugar. Stir in the rest of the ingredients one at a time in the order listed. Form the dough into a ball, wrap it in plastic wrap, and refrigerate it for at least two hours. Cut the dough into thirds. Roll each third ⅛-inch (5 mm) thick on a lightly floured board. Cut the dough into shapes with the cookie cutters. Place the cookies onto ungreased cookie sheets. Bake at 400° F (200° C) for 5 to 8 minutes.

**YIELD:** 100 small cookies
**EXCHANGE:** ½ fat
**CALORIES:** 29

# Pecan Tea Cookies

| | | |
|---|---|---|
| 2 cups | finely chopped pecans | 500 mL |
| 1 cup | margarine | 250 mL |
| 2 tablespoons | sugar | 30 mL |
| 2 packets | concentrated acesulfame-K | 2 packets |
| 2 cups | flour | 500 mL |
| 1 teaspoon | vanilla extract | 5 mL |
| 1 tablespoon | water | 15 mL |

Mix all the ingredients together. Chill for half an hour. Shape into small balls. Place on a cookie sheet coated with nonstick cooking spray. Bake in a 350° F (180° C) oven for 12 to 13 minutes until light brown.

**YIELD:**      80 cookies
**EXCHANGE:** 1 fat
**CALORIES:**  50

# Cinnamon Crescents

| | | |
|---|---|---|
| 1 cup | margarine or butter | 250 mL |
| 2 cups | flour, sifted | 500 mL |
| 1 | egg yolk | 1 |
| ¾ cup | nonfat sour cream | 190 mL |
| 3 tablespoons | sugar | 45 mL |
| 3 packets | concentrated acesulfame-K | 3 packets |
| ¾ cup | finely chopped walnuts | 190 mL |
| 2 teaspoons | cinnamon | 10 mL |

1 egg white, slightly beaten in 1 tablespoon (15 mL) water 1

Cut the margarine into the flour until the mixture resembles coarse crumbs. Stir in the egg yolk and sour cream. Form a ball. Cover with plastic wrap and chill for two hours. Combine the sugar, acesulfame-K, walnuts, and cinnamon. Diver the dough into fourths. Roll each into an 11-inch (28-cm) circle. Sprinkle each circle with a quarter of the sugar mixture. Cut into 16 wedges. Roll up the wedges, starting at the widest end. Place the rolls on an ungreased cookie sheet. Brush with egg white and water. Bake in a 350° F (180° C) oven for 20 minutes or until golden brown. Cool on wire racks.

**YIELD:**      48 cookies
**EXCHANGE:** ½ bread
                ½ fat
**CALORIES:**  70

# Snickerdoodles

| | | |
|---|---|---|
| 1 cup | margarine or butter | 250 mL |
| ¼ cup | sugar | 60 mL |
| 6 packets | concentrated acesulfame-K | 6 packets |
| 2 | eggs | 2 |
| 1 teaspoon | vanilla extract | 5 mL |
| 2⅔ cups | flour, sifted | 690 mL |
| 2 teaspoons | cream of tartar | 10 mL |
| 1 teaspoon | baking soda | 5 mL |

## COATING

| | | |
|---|---|---|
| 2 tablespoons | sugar | 30 mL |
| 1 teaspoon | cinnamon | 5 mL |

Beat the margarine until light. Add the sugar and acesul-fame-K and beat until fluffy. Beat in the eggs and vanilla. Sift together the flour, cream of tartar, and baking soda. Add this to the margarine mixture.

Combine the sugar and cinnamon in a separate bowl. With floured hands, shape the dough into small bols about 1 inch (2.5 cm) and roll each one in the sugar-cinnamon mixture. Place each 2 inches (5 cm) apart on an ungreased baking sheet. Bake at 400° F (200° C) for 8-10 minutes. Cool on wire racks.

| | |
|---|---|
| **YIELD:** | 6 dozen cookies |
| **EXCHANGE:** | ½ fat |
| **CALORIES:** | 44 |

# Peanut Butter Cookies

| 2 tablespoons | margarine or butter | 30 mL |
| ½ cup | peanut butter | 125 mL |
| ¼ cup | sugar | 60 mL |
| 3 packets | concentrated acesulfame-K | 3 packets |
| 1 | egg or egg substitute, beaten | 1 |
| 2 cups | flour | 500 mL |
| 4 teaspoons | baking powder | 20 mL |
| ⅓ cup | milk | 90 mL |

Cream the margarine thoroughly, add the peanut butter and cream together, then blend in the sugar and acesulfame-K. Add the beaten egg. Mix and sift the dry ingredients and add them alternately to the creamed mixture with the milk. Roll into small balls and place on a baking sheet coated with nonstick cooking spray. Flatten with the bottom of a glass dipped in flour. Then, using a fork, make criss-cross impressions in each cookie. Bake in a 400° F (200° C) oven for 7 minutes.

YIELD: 70 cookies
EXCHANGE: Free
CALORIES: 27

# Brownies

| | | |
|---|---|---|
| ½ cup | flour | 125 mL |
| ½ teaspoon | baking powder | 2 mL |
| ½ teaspoon | salt | 2 mL |
| 3 ounces | unsweetened chocolate (melted) | 90 g |
| ½ cup | shortening (soft) | 125 mL |
| 2 | eggs (beaten) | 2 |
| 2 tablespoons | granulated sugar | 30 mL |
| 1½ cups | sugar replacement | 375 mL |
| 1 teaspoon | vanilla extract | 5 mL |

Combine all ingredients. Beat vigorously until well blended. Spread mixture into greased 8-inch (20-cm) square pan. Bake at 350° F (175° C) for 30 to 35 minutes. Cut into 2-inch (5-cm) squares.

**MICROWAVE:** Cook on Medium for 8 to 10 minutes, or until puffed and dry on top. Cut into 2 inch (5-cm) squares.

**YIELD:** 16 brownies
**EXCHANGE 1 BROWNIE:** 1 ½ bread
1 ½ fat
**CALORIES 1 BROWNIE:** 136

# Cranberry Bars

| | | |
|---|---|---|
| 1¼ cups | flour | 300 mL |
| 1 cup | cereal crumbs | 250 mL |
| ¼ teaspoon | salt | 1 mL |
| ¼ cup | cold butter | 60 mL |
| 1 | egg (beaten) | 1 |
| 4 tablespoons | sugar replacement | 60 mL |
| 2 tablespoons | nuts | 30 mL |
| | vegetable cooking spray | |
| 1 | orange | 1 |
| 1½ cups | cranberries | 375 mL |
| 1/3 cup | water | 60 mL |
| 2 tablespoons | cornstarch | 30 mL |
| ½ teaspoon | ground allspice | 2 mL |

Combine flour, cereal crumbs, and salt in mixing bowl. Cut in cold butter until mixture resembles cornmeal. Combine egg and 1 tablespoon (15 mL) of the sugar replacement. Toss with fork until well blended. Combine 1 cup (250 mL) of the crumb mixture with nuts; reserve for topping. Press remaining crumb mixture into bottom of 8-inch (20-cm) square pan coated with vegetable cooking spray. Squeeze orange; reserve 1/3 cup (90 mL) of the juice. Grind the rest of the orange (except for seeds) with cranberries. Combine reserved orange juice, water, 3 tablespoons (45 mL) of the sugar replacement, cornstarch, and allspice. Stir in cranberry-orange mixture. Cook over medium heat until thick and clear, stirring frequently. Spread over crumb crust; sprinkle with reserved nut-crumb mixture. Bake at 350° F (175° C) for 25 minutes. Cool. Cut into 2-inch (5-cm) squares.

**YIELD:** 16 bars
**EXCHANGE 1 BAR:** 1 vegetable
1 fat
½ fruit
**CALORIES 1 BAR:** 92

# Blueberry Muffins

| | | |
|---|---|---|
| 1 ½ cups | flour          375 mL | |
| 1 ½ teaspoons | baking powder | 7 mL |
| ¼ teaspoon | baking soda | 1 mL |
| 1 tablespoon | canola oil 15 mL | |
| ⅓ cup | egg substitute | 90 mL |
| ½ cup | nonfat buttermilk | 125 mL |
| ½ teaspoon | vanilla extract | 2 mL |
| 2 tablespoons | nonfat sour cream | 30 mL |
| ¼ cup | apple juice concentrate | 60 mL |
| 1 cup | blueberries (fresh or frozen without sugar and defrosted) | 250 mL |
| 3 tablespoons | boiling water | 45 mL |
| 2 teaspoons | concentrated aspartame | 10 mL |

Sift together the flour, baking powder, and baking soda. Set aside. Use a wire whisk to combine the oil, egg substitute, buttermilk, vanilla extract, sour cream, and apple juice concentrate. Stir the flour mixture into the wet mixture. Do not overmix. Stir in the blueberries. Pour into a muffin tin that has been coated with nonstick cooking spray.

Bake in a preheated 375° F (190° C) oven for 30 minutes. As soon as the muffins are out of the oven, combine the boiling water and aspartame to make a glaze. Use a toothpick to make holes in the tops of the muffins. Use a pastry brush to cover the tops with the glaze.

**YIELD:** 12 muffins
**EXCHANGE:** 1 brad
**CALORIES:** 90

# PIES

## Basic Pie Shell

| | | |
|---|---|---|
| 1/3 cup | shortening | 90 mL |
| 1 cup | flour | 250 mL |
| ¼ teaspoon | salt | 1 mL |
| 2 to 4 tablespoons | ice water | 30 to 60 mL |

Chill shortening. Cut shortening into flour and salt until mixture forms crumbs. Add ice water, 1 tablespoon (15 mL) at a time. Flip mixture around in bowl until a ball forms. Wrap in plastic wrap. Chill at least 1 hour. Roll to fit 9-inch (23-cm) pie pan. Fill with pie filling or prick with fork. Bake at 425° F (220° C) for 10 to 12 minutes or until firm, or leave unbaked.

| | |
|---|---|
| **YIELD:** | 8 servings |
| **EXCHANGE 1 SERVING:** | 1 bread |
| | 2 fat |
| **CALORIES 1 SERVING:** | 170 |

## Apple Pie Filling for Pie or Tarts

| | | |
|---|---|---|
| 4 cups | apple, peeled, sliced thin | 1 L |
| 1 tablespoon | cinnamon | 15 mL |
| 1 teaspoon | nutmeg | 5 mL |
| 1 tablespoon | vanilla extract | 15 mL |
| 2 tablespoons | lemon juice | 30 mL |
| 6 packets | concentrated acesulfame-K | 6 packets |
| 1 teaspoon | grated lemon peel | 5 mL |

YIELD: 8 pie servings
EXCHANGE 1½ fruits
CALORIES: 89

# Washington's Cherry Pie

| | | |
|---|---|---|
| 9-inch | unbaked pie shell | 23-cm |
| 2 cups | unsweetened cherries | 500 mL |
| ¼ cup | soft margarine | 60 mL |
| 1 tablespoon | flour | 15 mL |
| ½ cup | sugar replacement | 125 mL |
| 2 | egg yolks | 2 |
| ¼ cup | evaporated milk | 60 mL |
| ½ teaspoon | vanilla extract | 2 mL |
| 2 | egg whites | 2 |
| 2 teaspoons | granulated sugar replacement | 10 mL |

Drain cherries; pour into unbaked pie shell. Cream margarine, flour, and sugar replacement. Add egg yolks and beat until smooth. Add evaporated milk and vanilla extract. Pour over cherries. Bake at 450° F (230° C) for 10 minutes. Reduce heat. Bake at 350° F (175° C) for 30 minutes. Whip egg whites until soft peaks form. Add granulated sugar; whip until thick and stiff. Top pie filling with meringue, carefully sealing edges. Bake at 350° F (175° C) for 12 to 15 minutes, or until delicately brown.

YIELD: 8 servings
EXCHANGE 1 SERVING: 1 fruit
1 fat
plus pie shell exchange
CALORIES 1 SERVING: 88
plus pie shell calories

# Fresh Strawberry Pie

| | | |
|---|---|---|
| 9-inch | baked pie shell | 23 cm |
| 5/8 oz. pkg. | lo-cal strawberry gelatin | 20-g pkg. |
| 1 quart | fresh strawberries | 1 L |
| 1 pkg. | lo-cal whipped topping (prepared) | 1 pkg. |

Prepare one envelope of gelatin as directed on package. Allow to semi-set. Rinse and hull berries; place in baked pie shell. Pour gelatin over top; chill until firm. Top with prepared whipped topping.

| | |
|---|---|
| **YIELD:** | 8 servings |
| **EXCHANGE 1 SERVING:** | ½ fruit |
| | plus pie shell exchange |
| **CALORIES 1 SERVING:** | 20 |
| | plus pie shell calories |

# Fine-Crumb Pie Shell

| | | |
|---|---|---|
| 1¼ cups | fine crumbs (graham cracker, dry cereal, Zwieback) | 300 mL |
| 3 tablespoons | margarine (melted) | 45 mL |
| 1 tablespoon | water | 15 mL |
| | spices (see spice and herb list) | |
| | sugar replacement | |

Combine crumbs with melted margarine and water; add spices and sugar replacement, if desired. Spread evenly in 9-inch (23 cm) pie pan. Press firmly onto sides and bottom. Either chill until set or bake at 325° F (165° C) for 8 to 10 minutes.

| **Yield:** | 8 servings |
| **Exchange 1 serving Graham Cracker:** | 1 bread |
| | 1 fat |
| **Calories 1 serving Graham Cracker:** | 85 |
| **Exchange 1 serving Dry Cereal:** | ½ bread |
| | 1 fat |
| **Calories 1 serving Dry Cereal:** | 64 |
| **Exchange 1 serving Zwieback:** | ½ bread |
| | 1 fat |
| **Calories 1 serving Zwieback:** | 70 |

# Blueberry Cream Pie

| 9-inch | baked pie shell | 23-cm |
| 2 cups | lo-cal whipped topping (prepared) | 500 mL |
| 1½ cups | Blueberry Topping (p. 161) | 375 mL |

Fold prepared whipped topping into Blueberry Topping. Spread into baked pie shell. Chill until firm.

| **Yield:** | 8 servings |
| **Exchange 1 serving:** | ½ fruit |
| | plus pie shell exchange |
| **Calories 1 serving:** | 30 |
| | plus pie shell calories |

# Cranberry-Pineapple Pie

| 9-inch | unbaked pie shell | 23-cm |
| 1½ cups | unsweetened crushed pineapple | 375 mL |
| ½ cup | sugar replacement | 125 mL |
| 1 tablespoon | cornstarch | 15 mL |
| ½ teaspoon | salt | 2 mL |
| 1 tablespoon | butter | 15 mL |
| 2 cups | cranberries | 500 mL |

Drain pineapple; reserve liquid. Blend ½ cup (125 mL) of the pineapple liquid with cornstarch. Cook until very thick. Stir in sugar replacement, salt and butter. Add cranberries and drained pineapple. Pour into unbaked pie shell. Bake at 425° F (220° C) for 30 to 40 minutes, or until set.

**YIELD:** 8 servings
**EXCHANGE 1 SERVING:** 1 fruit
½ fat
plus pie shell exchange
**CALORIES 1 SERVING:** 30
plus pie shell calories

# Strawberry Cream Pie

| | | |
|---|---|---|
| 9-inch | baked pie shell | 23-cm |
| 1 package | lo-cal vanilla pudding | 1 package |
| 1½ cups | Strawberry Topping (p. 161) | 375 mL |
| ¼ cup | fresh strawberries (halved) | 60 mL |
| 1 package | lo-cal whipped topping (prepared) | 1 package |

Prepare pudding as directed on package; cool slightly. Pour into baked pie shell. Cover with waxed paper; chill until set. Combine Strawberry Topping with fresh strawberries. Spread evenly on top of pudding. Top with prepared whipped topping.

**YIELD:** 8 servings
**EXCHANGE 1 SERVING:** 1 ½ fruit
½ milk
plus pie shell exchange
**CALORIES 1 SERVING:** 75
plus pie shell calories

# Lemon Cake Pie

| 9-inch | unbaked pie shell | 23-cm |
|---|---|---|
| ½ cup | sugar replacement | 125 mL |
| 2 tablespoons | flour | 30 mL |
| 2 tablespoons | margarine (soft) | 30 mL |
| 1 tablespoon | lemon rind | 15 mL |
| 3 tablespoons | lemon juice | 45 mL |
| 1 cup | skim milk | 250 mL |
| 2 | eggs, separated | 2 |

Combine sugar replacement, flour, margarine, lemon rind and juice, skim milk, and egg yolks. Beat vigorously. Fold in egg whites (well beaten). Pour into unbaked pie shell. Bake at 325° F (165° C) for 1 hour, or until set.

**YIELD:** 8 servings
**EXCHANGE 1 SERVING:** 1 milk
Plus pie shell exchange
**CALORIES 1 SERVING:** 40
Plus pie shell calories

# Fresh Rhubarb Pie

| 9-inch | unbaked pie shell | 23-cm |
|---|---|---|
| 1 quart | 1-inch (2.5-cm) pieces rhubarb | 1 L |
| 4 tablespoons | flour | 60 mL |
| ½ cup | sugar replacement | 125 mL |
| 2 | eggs (beaten) | 2 |

Mix rhubarb, flour, sugar replacement, and eggs. Pour into unbaked pie shell. Bake at 350° F (175° C) for 40 to 50 minutes, or until set.

| | |
|---|---|
| **YIELD:** | 8 servings |
| **EXCHANGE 1 SERVING:** | ½ fruit |
| | plus pie shell exchange |
| **CALORIES 1 SERVING:** | 68 |
| | plus pie shell calories |

# Strawberry Turnovers

| | | |
|---|---|---|
| ¼ teaspoon | cornstarch | 2 mL |
| 1 tablespoon | water | 15 mL |
| ½ cup | Strawberry Topping (p. 161) | 125 mL |
| 1 | dough for Basic Pie Shell (p. 188) | 1 |
| | Vanilla Gloss (p. 224) | |

Blend cornstarch and water. Add to Strawberry Topping. Cook over low heat until very thick. Roll pie dough thin. Cut into eight 4-inch (10-cm) squares. Place 1½ teaspoons (7 mL) of the strawberry mixture into center of each square. Fold each square into a triangle; press sides securely together to seal. Bake at 400° F (200° C) for 9 to 11 minutes, or until golden brown. Brush with Vanilla Gloss.

**MICROWAVE:** Use microwave only for strawberry filling. Blend cornstarch and water. Add to Strawberry Topping. Cook on High for 30 seconds, or until very thick. Proceed as above.

| | |
|---|---|
| **YIELD:** | 8 turnovers |
| **EXCHANGE 1 TURNOVER:** | 1 bread |
| **CALORIES 1 TURNOVER:** | 180 |

# FRUITS

## Apple-Go-Round

| | | |
|---|---|---|
| 1 | firm apple | 1 |
| ¼ cup | orange juice | 60 mL |
| 1 teaspoon | lemon juice | 5 mL |
| 1 tablespoon | raisins | 15 mL |
| 1 tablespoon | celery (diced) | 15 mL |
| 2 tablespoons | applesauce | 30 mL |
| | lettuce leaf | |

Slice off top of apple; remove core. Prick outside with sharp fork. Place apple in tall narrow bowl. Combine orange and lemon juice; pour over apple. (Add extra water if apple is not covered.) Marinate in refrigerator 4 to 5 hours. Combine raisins, celery, and applesauce. Allow to mellow at room temperature 2 hours. Chill thoroughly. Drain apple. Cut apple into 8 sections, slicing almost to the bottom. Fill with applesauce mixture. Place on crisp lettuce leaf.

**YIELD:** 1 serving
**EXCHANGE:** 2 fruit
**CALORIES:** 54

# Baked Apple Dumpling

| 1 teaspoon | raisins | 5 mL |
| 2 tablespoons | orange juice | 30 mL |
| ½ teaspoon | sugar replacement | 3 mL |
| 1 small | apple | 1 small |
| | biscuit dough for 1 biscuit | |

Combine raisins and orange juice in saucepan. Heat to a boil. Add sugar replacement. Cover. Allow to rest while preparing remaining ingredients. Core apple; with a fork or toothpick, prick the inside of the apple cavity. On floured board, roll biscuit dough very thin and large enough to wrap around apple. Place apple in center of dough. Fill apple cavity with raisin mixture. Wrap dough around apple and secure at top. Place in baking dish. Bake at 375° F (190° C) for 25 to 30 minutes.

**YIELD:** 1 serving
**EXCHANGE:** 1 bread
1 fruit
**CALORIES:** 142

# Sweet 'n' Sour Strawberries

| 2 cups | fresh or frozen strawberries with no sugar added | 500 mL |
| 3 packets | concentrated acesulfame-K | 3 packets |
| 2 tablespoons | balsamic vinegar | 30 mL |

Slice the strawberries in half. Sprinkle them with acesulfame-K and vinegar. Stir to combine. This is best served chilled, and is a real "company" dessert when presented in fancy glasses.

**YIELD:** 4 servings  **CALORIES:** 24
**EXCHANGE:** Free

# Apple Crisp

| | | |
|---|---|---|
| 4 cups | apples, sliced | 1 L |
| ¼ cup | water | 60 mL |
| 1 tablespoon | molasses | 15 mL |
| 3 packets | concentrated acesulfame-K | 3 packets |
| 1 tablespoon | lemon juice | 15 mL |
| 1 teaspoon | cinnamon | 5 mL |
| ¼ teaspoon | cloves | 1 mL |
| ¾ cup | oatmeal | 190 mL |
| 2 teaspoons | margarine or butter | 10 mL |
| 2 packets | concentrated acesulfame-K | 2 packets |

Combine the apples, water, molasses, 3 packets of acesul-fame-K, lemon juice, cinnamon, and cloves. Mix well. Arrange the apple mixture in an 8-inch (20 cm) square baking dish coated with non-stick cooking spray. Combine the remaining ingredients and sprinkle the mixture over the apples. Bake at 375° F (190° C) for 30 minutes or until the apples are tender and the topping is lightly browned.

YIELD:     8 servings
EXCHANGE: 1 bread
CALORIES:  84

# Peach Melba

| | | |
|---|---|---|
| ½ cup | raspberries | 125 mL |
| ½ teaspoon | sugar replacement | 5 mL |
| ½ cup | dietetic vanilla ice cream | 125 mL |
| ½ | peach (sliced) | ½ |

Slightly mash raspberries and sugar replacement. Allow to rest 5 minutes. Place ice cream in dish. Top with peach slices and raspberries.

**YIELD:** 1 serving
**EXCHANGE:** 1 bread
1 fruit
**CALORIES:** 120

# Nectarine Purée

| 3 fresh, sweet | nectarines | 3 |
| 2 teaspoons | lemon juice | 10 mL |
| 2 teaspoons | concentrated aspartame | 10 mL |

Drop the nectarines into a large pan of boiling water. Turn off the heat. Let stand for one minute to loosen the skins. Drain the hot water; then pour cold water over the fruit and slip off their skins. Place the nectarines in a food processor or blender with the lemon juice and aspartame. The amount of aspartame will vary, depending on the tartness of the fruit. Purée. Spoon into glass dessert dishes.

**YIELD:** 3 servings
**EXCHANGE:** 1 fruit
**CALORIES:** 68

# Browned Bananas

| 1 | banana, peeled | 1 |

Slice the banana in half lengthwise. Place it on a broiler pan that has been coated with non-stick cooking spray. Place the pan under a preheated broiler a few inches from the heat. Watch it carefully and remove the tray from the oven as the banana becomes browned and bubbly. Serve hot. A small dollop of sugar-free, frozen nonfat vanilla yogurt makes a nice garnish for this dessert.

YIELD: 2 servings
EXCHANGE: 1 fruit
CALORIES: 53

# Poached Pears and Raspberries

| 6 | medium pears | 6 |
|---|---|---|
| 1 packet | concentrated acesulfame-K, | 1 packet |
| or | | |
| 1 tablespoon | sugar | (15 mL) |
| ¼ cup | water | 60 mL |
| 1-inch | piece of vanilla bean, slit | 2.5 cm |
| 2 cups | raspberries, fresh or | |
| | frozen, unsweetened | 500 mL |
| 2 tablespoons | fruit-only, seedless raspberry jam | 30 mL |

Peel, core, and halve the pears. Combine the acesulfame (or sugar) and water in a saucepan and bring to a boil. Reduce the heat to low and add the vanilla bean and pear halves. Cover. Simmer for 5 minutes or so, until the pears are fork-tender. Cool. Drain. In a small bowl, gently toss the raspberries and jelly. Put two pear halves on each serving plate. Mound the raspberries on top of the pears.

YIELD: 6 servings
EXCHANGE: 2 fruits
CALORIES: 168

# Four-Fruit Compote

| | | |
|---|---|---|
| 1 | large orange | 1 |
| 1 | small cantaloupe | 1 |
| ½ pound | seedless grapes | 225 g |
| 3 | ripe pears | 3 |
| ½ cup | water | 125 mL |
| 3 tablespoons | lemon juice | 45 mL |
| 3 packets | concentrated acesulfame-K | 3 packets |
| ¼ teaspoon | mace | 1 mL |
| 2 tablespoons | rum (optional) | 30 mL |

Cut the orange into segments, remove the membrane, and put the segments into a large bowl. Peel the cantaloupe, cut it cross-wise and remove the seeds. Cut into large cubes. Add the cubes and the stemmed grapes to the oranges. Core the pears, then cut them into large cubes. Sprinkle the pear cubes with lemon juice and add them to the fruit bowl. Mix together the water, lemon juice, acesulfame-K, and mace. Add rum, if desired. Cover; refrigerate for an hour or more before serving.

**YIELD:** 8 servings
**EXCHANGE:** 1 fruit
**CALORIES:** 76

# Mixed-Berry Smoothie

| | | |
|---|---|---|
| 12-ounce-can | evaporated nonfat milk | 354 mL-can |
| 1 tablespoon | cornstarch | 15 mL |
| 3 packets | concentrated acesulfame-K | 3 packets |
| 1 teaspoon | almond extract | 5 mL |
| 1 teaspoon | concentrated aspartame | 5 mL |
| 12-ounce-bag | frozen mixed berries | 340 g-bag |
| 2 cups | nonfat yogurt, no sugar added (plain or vanilla) | 500 mL |

Combine the first three ingredients and stir them together in a saucepan. Heat just to a boil, then reduce the heat and simmer for 5 minutes or until the sauce thickens, stir constantly with a wire whisk. Turn off the heat; stiring in the almond extract, aspartame, and berries. Let cool and then fold in the yogurt.

**YIELD:** 8 servings
**EXCHANGE:** 1 milk
**CALORIES:** 99

# Ambrosia

| | | |
|---|---|---|
| 2 | oranges, peeled with membrane removed | 2 |
| 2 teaspoons | measures-like-sugar aspartame | 10 mL |
| 2 | bananas, peeled | 2 |
| ¼ cup | shredded coconut | 125 mL |

Slice the oranges and bananas thin. Place a layer of orange slices in the bottom of a serving bowl. Sprinkle with some of the aspartame. Place a layer of bananas over the oranges, then a layer of coconut. Make many layers of fruit, ending with a layer of coconut. Cover with plastic wrap; refrigerate for at least an hour before serving.

**YIELD:** 4 servings
**EXCHANGE:** 1½ fruit
**CALORIES:** 84

# PUDDINGS, CUSTARDS, AND GELATINS

## Rhubarb Pudding

| | | |
|---|---|---|
| 1 quart | rhubarb (cut in pieces) | 1 L |
| 1 cup | water | 250 mL |
| 2 tablespoons | cornstarch | 30 mL |
| 1 teaspoon | sugar replacement | 5 mL |

Cut rhubarb into pieces. Place rhubarb in saucepan. Add the water. Cook rhubarb until tender. Mix cornstarch with small amount of cold water; add to rhubarb. Cook until thickened. Remove from heat; add sugar replacement. Stir until dissolved.

**MICROWAVE:** Place rhubarb in large bowl. Add the water. Cook on High for 4 minutes, or until tender. Mix cornstarch with small amount of cold water; add to rhubarb. Cook on High for 1 to 2 minutes, or until thickened.

| | |
|---|---|
| **YIELD:** | 6 servings |
| **EXCHANGE 1 SERVING:** | 1/8 fruit |
| | 1/8 bread |
| **CALORIES 1 SERVING:** | 22 |

# Raisin Rice Pudding

| 1 package | lo-cal rice pudding | 1 package |
| ½ cup | raisins | 125 mL |

Prepare rice pudding as directed on package. Soak raisins in warm water for 1 hour. Drain thoroughly. Add raisins to rice pudding.

**YIELD:** 5 servings, ½ cup (125 mL each)
**EXCHANGE 1 SERVING:** ½ bread
½ milk
½ fruit
**CALORIES 1 SERVING:** 100

# Bread Pudding

| ½ loaf | "light" sourdough bread | ½ loaf |
| 12-ounce can | evaporated skim milk | 375-mL can |
| ½ cup | unsweetened applesauce | 125 mL |
| 1 teaspoon | vanilla extract | 5 mL |
| ½ cup | skim milk | 125 mL |
| 8 packets | acesulfame-K | 8 packets |
| ⅓ cup | raisins | 90 mL |
| ½ teaspoon | cinnamon | 2 mL |
| 4 | egg whites | 4 |

Cut the bread slices into cubes; place them on a cookie sheet coated with non-stick cooking spray. Place the tray in a pre-heated 350° F (180° C) oven for 10 minutes. Combine all the other ingredients and add the bead. Toss well and place in an ovenproof baking dish that has been sprayed with non-stick vegetable cooking spray. Place this baking dish in a large pan of water filled nearly to the top of the baking dish, and place the pan in a preheated 350° F (180° C) oven. Bake for 40 minutes. Serve hot or cold.

**YIELD:** 8 servings
**EXCHANGE:** 1 ½ bread
**CALORIES:** 109

# Baked Custard

| | | |
|---|---|---|
| 12-ounce can | evaporated skim milk | 375-mL can |
| 2 packets | acesulfame-K | 2 packets |
| 1 teaspoon | sugar | 5 mL |
| 1 teaspoon | lemon peel | 5 mL |
| 1 teaspoon | margarine or butter | 5 mL |
| ¼ cup | egg substitute | 60 mL |
| 1 teaspoon | vanilla extract | 5 mL |
| sprinkling | nutmeg (optional) | sprinkling |

Heat the milk over hot water in the top of a double boiler. Add the acesulfame-K, sugar, lemon peel, and margarine and whisk together for a few minutes. In a separate bowl, use an electric mixer to beat the egg substitute for a few minutes until foamy and light. Add a little hot milk mixture to the beaten egg substitute and beat. Gradually pour in the rest of the hot milk and beat constantly. Add the vanilla extract and heat briefly. Pour into small ovenproof custard dishes that have been coated with non-stick cooking spray. If desired, sprinkle the top with nutmeg. Place the small cups in a larger pan of hot water. Bake in a preheated 325° F (160° C) oven for approximately 40 minutes. A knife inserted in the center should come out clean. Chill before serving.

**YIELD:** 4 servings
**EXCHANGE:** 1 milk
**CALORIES:** 97

# Tapioca Pudding

| | | |
|---|---|---|
| 3 cups | skim milk | 750 mL |
| ¼ cup | quick-cooking (instant) tapioca | 125 mL |
| ¼ teaspoon | salt (optional) | 1 mL |
| ¼ cup | egg substitute | 60 mL |
| 1 | egg white, beaten | 1 |
| 1 teaspoon | vanilla extract | 5 mL |
| 2 ½ teaspoons | concentrated aspartame | 7 mL |

Whisk together the milk, tapioca, salt (optional), egg substitute, and beaten egg white in the top of a double boiler. Heat the water in the lower part to boiling. Cover the top part and cook for five minutes while stirring. Remove from the heat; add the vanilla extract and aspartame. The pudding will thicken as it cools.

**YIELD:** 6 servings
**EXCHANGE:** 1 bread
**CALORIES:** 79

# Pineapple Mousse

| | | |
|---|---|---|
| 20-ounce can | pineapple, packed in juice, drained | 625-mL can |
| 2 tablespoons | fructose | 30 mL |
| 1 cup | evaporated skim milk, chilled | 250 mL |
| 1 envelope | unflavored gelatin | 1 envelope |
| 1 tablespoon | lemon juice | 15 mL |

Puree the pineapple in a blender or food processor. Add the fructose; stir. Set aside. In a mixing bowl, whip the evaporated milk until thick and creamy. In the top of a double boiler, sprinkle the gelatin over the lemon juice. Let stand 3 to 5 minutes. Stir over hot water until dissolved. Stir the gelatin into the whipped milk. Fold the pineapple mixture into the milk. Spoon into dessert dishes. Chill until set.

**YIELD:** 16 servings
**EXCHANGE:** 1 milk
**CALORIES:** 51

# Chocolate Pudding

| ¼ cup | sugar | 60 mL |
| 3 packets | concentrated acesulfame-K | 3 packets |
| 2 tablespoons | unsweetened cocoa powder | 30 mL |
| 3 tablespoons | cornstarch | 45 mL |
| 2 cups | nonfat milk | 500 mL |
| 1 teaspoon | vanilla extract | 5 mL |

Combine the sugar, acesulfame-K, cocoa, and cornstarch in a saucepan. Add about ½ cup (125 mL) milk. Stir with a wire whisk until dissolved and the mixture is smooth. Add the remaining milk and vanilla extract. Cook, stirring occasionally until thick, about 5 minutes. Cool before serving.

**YIELD:** 4 servings
**EXCHANGE:** 1 bread
         ½ fruit
**CALORIES:** 118

# Lemon Pudding

| 1 envelope | unflavored gelatin, unsweetened | 1 envelope |
| 2 tablespoons | cold water | 30 mL |
| ½ cup | boiling water | 125 mL |
| 1½ cups | nonfat buttermilk | 375 mL |
| 2 teaspoons | lemon rind | 10 mL |
| 2 teaspoons | lemon juice | 10 mL |
| 2 teaspoons | concentrated aspartame | 10 mL |
| 2 drops | yellow food coloring (optional) | 2 drops |

In a large mixing bowl, sprinkle the gelatin over the cold water to soften. Let sit for a few minutes. Pour the boiling water over it and stir until completely dissolved. Add the remaining ingredients and whisk together. Pour into five individual pudding dishes that have been sprayed very lightly with non-stick cooking spray. The pudding may be served in the individual dishes or unmoulded onto separate plates. This pudding can be served plain or dressed up with a little fresh fruit or a plain, frozen strawberry.

**YIELD:** 5 servings
**EXCHANGE:** ½ milk
**CALORIES:** 31

# Black Cherry Gelatin

| | | |
|---|---|---|
| 1 envelope | flavored gelatin | 1 envelope |
| ¼ cup | cold water | 60 mL |
| 2 packets | concentrated acesulfame-K | 2 packets |
| 2 cups | sugar-free black cherry soda | 500 mL |

Sprinkle the gelatin over the water in the top of a double boiler. Let stand for 5 minutes. Meanwhile, in another bowl, combine the remaining ingredients. Stir the gelatin over hot water until dissolved. Pour into the black cherry mixture. Chill until set. Garnish with fresh fruit slices if desired.

**YIELD:** 4 servings
**EXCHANGE:** negligable
**CALORIES:** 7

# Jell Jells

| | | |
|---|---|---|
| 1 quart | lo-cal orange soda | 1 L |
| 4 envelopes | unflavored gelatin | 4 envelopes |
| 1½ pkg. | lo-cal orange gelatin | 1½ pkg. |

Bring orange soda to a boil. Combine gelatins together in large bowl; add boiling water. Stir to dissolve. Pour into a pan. Chill until firm. Cut into cubes.

**EXCHANGE:** Negligible
**CALORIES:** Negligible

# Homemade Ice Cream

| | | |
|---|---|---|
| 13-ounce can | evaporated milk | 385-mL can |
| 2 tablespoons | sugar replacement | 30 mL |
| 1 ½ cups | whole milk | 375 mL |
| 1 tablespoon | vanilla extract | 15 mL |
| 3 | eggs (well beaten) | 3 |

Combine evaporated milk and sugar replacement. Beat well until sugar is dissolved. Add whole milk and vanilla extract; beat well. Add eggs; beat eggs into milk mixture vigorously. Pour into ice cream maker. Freeze according to manufacturer's directions.

**YIELD:** 8 servings
**EXCHANGE 1 SERVING:** ½ milk
½ lean meat
**CALORIES 1 SERVING:** 122

# Lemon Ice Freeze

| | | |
|---|---|---|
| 1 envelope | unflavored gelatin | 1 envelope |
| 1½ cups | milk | 375 mL |
| 2 | egg yolks (slightly beaten) | 2 |
| ¼ teaspoon | salt | 2 mL |
| ½ cup | sugar replacement | 125 mL |
| 2 teaspoons | lemon extract | 10 mL |
| 2 tablespoons | lemon peel | 30 mL |
| 2 | egg whites (stiffly beaten) | 2 |

Soften gelatin in ¼ cup (60 mL) of the milk; set aside. Combine egg yolks, remaining milk, salt, sugar replacement, lemon extract and peel in top of double boiler. Cook until thick and creamy. Remove from heat. Add gelatin mixture; stir until dissolved. Cool. Pour into ice cube tray and freeze. Place mixture in cold bowl and beat until smooth; fold in stiffly beaten egg whites. Return to tray and refreeze.

**YIELD:** 6 servings
**EXCHANGE 1 SERVING:** ½ milk exchange
⅓ meat
**CALORIES 1 SERVING:** 100

# Frozen Strawberry Yogurt

| | | |
|---|---|---|
| 8-ounce pkg. | frozen strawberries, no sugar added | 226-g pkg. |
| 1½ teaspoons | lemon juice | 7 mL |
| 2 teaspoons | aspartame | 10 mL |
| 1 tablespoon | vanilla extract | 15 mL |
| 1½ cups | nonfat yogurt, no sugar added (plain or vanilla) | 375 mL |

Put fruit in food processor with flavorings. Puree; add yogurt. Freeze in small yogurt containers for easy serving.

**YIELD:** 6 servings
**EXCHANGE:** 1 milk
**CALORIES:** 76

# Banana Sherbet

| 1 cup | nonfat, sugar-free | |
| | banana-cream-pie-flavored yogurt | 250 mL |
| 1 cup | mashed bananas | 250 mL |
| 1 teaspoon | concentrated aspartame | 5 mL |
| 1 teaspoon | vanilla extract | 5 mL |
| ½ teaspoon | banana extract | 2mL |

Combine all the ingredients in a food processor. Pour into two small yogurt containers; freeze for a few hours or overnight.

**YIELD:** 4 servings
**EXCHANGE:** 1 fruit
          ½ milk
**CALORIES:** 104

# Frosty Frozen Dessert

| 1 | egg white | 1 |
| ⅓ cup | water | 90 mL |
| ⅓ cup | nonfat dry milk | 90 mL |
| ⅓ cup | egg substitute | 90 mL |
| ⅓ cup | measures-like-sugar aspartame | 90 mL |
| ¾ cup | fruit purée such as nectarines | 180 mL |

Use an electric mixer to beat together the first three ingredients until a stiff mixture forms. Set aside. Take a separate mixing bowl and beat together the remaining ingredients until smooth. Put the bowl of beaten egg whites back under the beaters, then gently beat the fruit-and-egg-substitute mixture into the beaten egg whites. Pour into small yogurt containers and freeze for several hours or overnight.

**YIELD:** 11 servings, ½ cup (125 mL) each
**EXCHANGE:** ½ milk
**CALORIES:** 36

# Icy Grapes

Wash the grapes and place them in the freezer for several hours or overnight. Serve in fancy wine glasses.

For ½ cup (125 mL) grapes:
**EXCHANGE:** 1 fruit
**CALORIES:** 54

# DESSERTS FOR SPECIAL OCCASIONS

## Grand Marnier Soufflé for Six

| | | |
|---|---|---|
| 2 tablespoons | margarine or butter | 30 mL |
| 2½ tablespoons | regular all-purpose flour | 37 mL |
| ¾ cup | skim milk | 190 mL |
| 1 packet | concentrated acesulfame-K | 1 packet |
| 2 | egg yolks, beaten | 2 |
| 3 | egg whites | 3 |
| ⅛ teaspoon | cream of tartar | 0.5 mL |
| 3 tablespoons | Grand Marnier | 45 mL |

In a saucepan, melt the margarine or butter and remove it from the heat. Stir in the flour and milk; cook, stirring over medium heat, until thickened and smooth. Stir in the acesulfame-K; cool slightly; add egg yolks.

In a medium bowl, beat the egg whites until foamy; add the cream of tartar, beating until stiff peaks form when the beater is raised. Gently fold the egg yolk mixture and Grand Marnier into the egg whites. Turn into a one-quart soufflé dish or casserole coated with non-stick cooking spray. Bake for 10 minutes in a preheated 450° F (230° C) oven, then turn down the heat to 325° F (160° C) and bake 15 minutes longer. Serve immediately.

# Hot Apple Soufflé

| ½ cup | margarine or butter | 125 mL |
| ½ cup | flour | 125mL |
| 2 cups | cold skim milk | 500 mL |
| 2 tablespoons | granulated sugar | 30 mL |
| 1 packet | concentrated acesulfame K | 1 packet |
| | grated peel from ½ lemon | |
| 2 medium | apples | 2 |
| 4 | eggs, separated | 4 |
| 2 tablespoons | slivered toasted almonds | 30 mL |

About 2¼ hours before serving, melt the margarine in a medium saucepan; stir in the flour, then the milk. Cook, stirring constantly, until smooth and thickened. Blend in the sugar, acesulfame-K, and lemon peel; let cool slightly, stirring occasionally.

Meanwhile, wash, pare, and core the apples, then cut each into about 10 lengthwise wedges. Arrange them evenly over the bottom of a 2-quart (2 L) casserole. Beat the egg whites until stiff. Blend the yolks into the flour-milk mixture, then carefully fold in the egg whites. Pour this mixture over the apples, then sprinkle it with almonds. Bake in a preheated 325° F (160° C) oven for 1¼ hours or until light brown and firm. Serve at once.

**YIELD:** 8 servings
**EXCHANGE:** 1 bread
½ meat
1 fat
**CALORIES:** 229

# Chocolate Soufflé

| | | |
|---|---|---|
| ½ cup | unsweetened cocoa powder | 125 mL |
| 2 tablespoons | powdered sugar | 30 mL |
| ½ cup | measures-like-sugar saccharin | 125 mL |
| 7 packets | concentrated acesulfame-K | 7 packets |
| 2 tablespoons | cornstarch | 30 mL |
| dash | salt (optional) | dash |
| ½ cup | nonfat milk | 125 mL |
| ½ cup | water | 125 mL |
| 4 | egg whites | 4 |
| ½ teaspoon | cream of tartar | 2 mL |
| ¼ cup | egg substitute | 60 mL |
| 1 teaspoon | vanilla extract | 5 mL |
| 2 tablespoons | measures-like-sugar aspartame | 30 mL |

Sift the cocoa, sugar, saccharin, acesulfame-K, salt, and cornstarch together twice. Put them in the top of a double boiler and add the nonfat milk and water. Whisk constantly while cooking until the mixture is smooth and thick, about eight minutes. Remove from the heat. Beat the egg whites with an electric mixer until they hold their shape; add the cream of tartar and continue beating until stiff peaks form. Pour the egg substitute and vanilla extract into the chocolate mixture. Mix. Add a small amount of the beaten egg whites into the chocolate mixture to lighten. Then use a rubber spatula to fold in the rest of the egg whites.

Pour into a 6 cup (1.5 L) soufflé dish that has been coated with nonstick cooking spray. Bake in a preheated 400° F (200° C) oven for 20 minutes. Do not overcook; the center will be a little runny to make a sauce. As soon as the soufflé is out of the oven, dust aspartame over the top.

**YIELD:** 8 servings
**EXCHANGE:** ½ bead
**CALORIES:** 54

# Fruit Trifle

Trifles are usually served in large, straight-sided, clear-glass pedestal bowls. A traditional trifle consists of layers of brandy-soaked cake, fruit, pudding, and whipped cream. Trifles look beautiful and are delicious. When you're serving a crowd, a trifle is sure to please.

To assemble a trifle, use angel food cake, hot-milk sponge cake, or yellow cake. Recipes for these cakes are in the Cake section. Tear the cake into 2 x 2-inch (5 x 5 cm) bits and spread some on the bottom of the trifle bowl. Drop on a layer of sugar-free vanilla pudding, then add a layer of fruit. Blueberries, kiwis, and strawberries make an attractive and delicious combination. Then add a layer of sugar-free whipped topping. After the topping layer, start again with cake. Make as many layers as you have ingredients and room in the dish. Or, make individual trifles with pudding, fruit, topping, and a bit of leftover cake. Assemble the layers in wine or champagne glasses for a festive look.

Here are a few tips to make trifles suitable for people on diabetic diets:

• Most "low-sugar/low-fat" whipped toppings dissolve after half an hour or so. That means you need to assemble the trifle close to serving time.

• Use only ingredients that you know are suitable. Stay away from frozen or canned puddings or fruit with sugar.

• Bananas need to be tossed in lemon juice if you're using banana slices. Otherwise, they turn dark, gooey, and unappetizing.

• Traditional trifle recipes call for cake soaked in brandy or other liqueur. We leave that out and instead add brandy extract to the pudding.

# Cream Puffs

## The puff pastry

| | | |
|---|---|---|
| 1 cup | water | 250 mL |
| ⅓ cup | canola oil | 90 mL |
| 1 cup | flour | 250 mL |
| 4 | eggs or equivalent egg substitute | 4 |
| 1 teaspoon | butter-flavored extract | 5 mL |
| 1 teaspoon | vanilla extract | 5 mL |

Heat the water and oil to rolling boil. Lower the heat and add the flour all at once, stirring with a wooden spoon until mixture forms a ball. Remove from the heat. With an electric mixer, beat in the eggs thoroughly, one at a time. Add the butter-flavored extract. Using a spoon, drop 12 cream puffs onto ungreased cookie sheets. Bake in a 400° F (200° C) oven for 10 minutes. Reduce the heat to 350° F (180° C) and bake for 25 minutes longer. Do not remove the cream puffs from the oven until they are quite firm to the touch. Cool the shells away from drafts before filling. To fill, cut horizontally using a sharp knife. If any damp dough remains inside, scoop it out before filling.

Fill the shells with pudding. Top with whipped topping and Chocolate Sauce.

**YIELD:** 12 cream puffs
**EXCHANGE:** ½ bread
1 fat
**CALORIES:** 101

# Crepes

This recipe makes 14 five-inch (13 cm) crepes. You can make them in a larger skillet and use strawberry or blueberry topping or a different fruit filling such as fruit-only jam.

| | | |
|---|---|---|
| 1 packet | concentrated acesulfame-K | 1 packet |
| 1 cup | skim milk | 250 mL |
| 2 tablespoons | safflower oil | 30 mL |
| ½ cup | egg substitute | 125 mL |
| ½ cup | flour | 125 mL |
| 2 teaspoons | baking powder | 10 mL |
| ¼ teaspoon | vanilla extract | 1 mL |

Combine all the ingredients in a blender and blend for a minute or so or mix with an electric mixer until the batter is smooth. Heat a small, oiled skillet or crepe pan until a drop of water "dances" when you splash it on the hot surface. Add 1/3 cup (90 mL) of the batter and move the pan around so the batter covers evenly. Cook over medium heat on one side until the edges are browned and there are bubbles throughout the crepe. Turn and cook on the other side to brown. Spoon one tablespoon (15 mL) of Strawberry Topping on each crepe and roll the crepes up. Top with a dollop of your favorite whipped topping.

YIELD:       14 Crepes, 5 inches (13 cm)
EXCHANGE: ½ fat
CALORIES:   44
Plus calories and exchanges for filling and topping

# Crepes Suzettes Sauce

| | | |
|---|---|---|
| ¾ cup | orange juice | 190 mL |
| 1 teaspoon | grated orange peel | 5 mL |
| 1½ teaspoons | cornstarch | 7 mL |
| 1 packet | concentrated acesulfame-K | 1 packet |
| 1 teaspoon | margarine or butter | 5 mL |
| 1 teaspoon | concentrated aspartame | 5 mL |
| ½ teaspoon | orange extract (use 1 teaspoon [2 mL] if liqueur is omitted) | 2 mL |
| 2 tablespoons | orange-flavored liqueur, such as Grand Marnier | 30 mL |

In a saucepan whisk together the orange juice, orange peel, cornstarch, and acesulfame-K. Heat to boiling, then immediately reduce the heat and cook over a medium flame, stirring constantly. When the mixture is thickened, turn off the heat.

Stir in the margarine, aspartame, orange extract, and liqueur if desired. Take each crepe and fold in half, then again, and arrange on a separate plate. Spoon a little crepes suzettes sauce over each.

**YIELD:** 6 servings
**EXCHANGE:** Negligible
**CALORIES:** 22

# CANDY

## Fudge Candy

| | | |
|---|---|---|
| 13-ounce can | evaporated milk | 385-ml can |
| 3 tablespoons | cocoa | 45 mL |
| ¼ cup | butter | 60 mL |
| 1 tablespoons | sugar replacement | 15 mL |
| dash | salt | dash |
| 1 teaspoon | vanilla extract | 5mL |
| 2½ cups | unsweetened cereal crumbs | 625 mL |
| ¼ cup | nuts (very finely chopped) | 60 mL |

Combine milk and cocoa in saucepan; cook and beat over low heat until cocoa is dissolved. Add butter, sugar replacement, salt, and vanilla. Bring to a boil; reduce heat and cook for 2 minutes. Remove from heat; add cereal crumbs and work in with wooden spoon. Cool 15 minutes. Divide in half; roll each half into a tube, 8 inches (20 cm) long. Roll each tube in finely chopped nuts. Wrap in waxed paper; chill overnight. Cut into ¼-inch (6-mm) slices.

**YIELD:** 64 slices
**EXCHANGE 2 SLICES:** ½ bread
½ fat
**CALORIES 2 SLICES:** 60

# Chocolate Butter Creams

| | | |
|---|---|---|
| 3-oz. pkg. | cream cheese (softened) | 90-g pkg. |
| 2 T. | skim milk | 30 mL |
| 1½ T. | white vanilla extract | 7 mL |
| 1 cup | powdered sugar replacement | 250 mL |
| 1 recipe | Chocolate Topping (p. 224) | 1 recipe |

Beat cream cheese, milk and vanilla until fluffy; stir in powdered sugar replacement. Form into 30 balls and dip each one in chocolate.

**YIELD:** 30 creams
**EXCHANGE 1 CREAM:** ¼ low-fat milk
**CALORIES 1 CREAM:** 31

# Chocolate Crunch Candy

| | | |
|---|---|---|
| 1 cup | nonfat dry milk powder | 250 mL |
| ½ cup | cocoa | 125 mL |
| 2 tablespoons | liquid fructose | 30 mL |
| 3 tablespoons | water | 45 mL |
| 1 ½ cups | chow mein noodles | 375 mL |

Combine milk powder and cocoa in food processor or blender, blending to a fine powder. Stir in fructose and water and beat until smooth and creamy. Slightly crush the chow mein noodles and fold them into chocolate mixture. Drop by teaspoonfuls onto waxed paper. Cool at room temperature.

**YIELD:** 30 pieces
**EXCHANGE 1 PIECE:** 1/5 bread
**CALORIES 1 PIECE:** 11

# Butter Sticks

| | | |
|---|---|---|
| 7 large | shredded wheat biscuits | 7 large |
| ½ cup | crunchy peanut butter | 125 mL |
| 3 T. | granulated sugar replacement | 45 mL |
| 2 | egg whites | 2 |
| 1 T. | flour | 15 mL |
| 1 T. | water | 15 mL |
| 1 T. | baking powder | 5 mL |
| 1 t. | vanilla extract | 5 mL |
| 1 recipe | Chocolate Topping (p. 224) | 1 recipe |

Break biscuits into large bowl or food processor. Add peanut butter, sugar replacement, egg whites, flour, water, baking powder and vanilla. Work with wooden spoon or steel blade until mixture is completely blended; mixture will be sticky. Form into 16 sticks and place them on an ungreased cookie sheet. Bake at 400° F (200° C) for 10 minutes, or until surface feels hard. Remove; cool slightly. Dip in chocolate.

**YIELD:** 16 sticks
**EXCHANGE 1 STICK:** 2/3 bread
**CALORIES 1 STICK:** 115

# Sugared Pecans

| | | |
|---|---|---|
| ½ cup | water | 250 mL |
| ¼ cup | granulated sugar replacement | 60 mL |
| ¼ cup | granulated brown sugar replacement | 60 mL |
| 1 cup | pecan halves | 250 mL |

Combine water and sugar replacements in saucepan, stirring to dissolve. Bring to boil, and boil for 3 minutes. Stir in pecans until completely coated; remove pan from heat. Allow pecans to rest in sugar water for 2 to 3 minutes. Remove with slotted spoon and cool completely.

YIELD:      1 cup (250 mL)
EXCHANGE 1 SERVING:   1 fat
CALORIES 1 SERVING:   48

# Cookie Brittle

| ½ cup | margarine | 125 mL |
| 2 teaspoons | vanilla extract | 10 mL |
| 1 teaspoon | salt | 5 mL |
| 3 tablespoons | granulated sugar replacement | 45 mL |
| 2 cups | flour (sifted) | 500 mL |
| 1 cup | semisweet chocolate chips | 250 mL |
| ½ cup | walnuts (chopped fine) | 125 mL |

Combine margarine, vanilla, salt and sugar replacement in mixing bowl or food processor; beat until smooth. Stir in flour, chocolate chips and walnuts. Press into ungreased 15 x 10-inch (39 x 25-cm) pan. Bake at 375° F (190° C) for 25 minutes. Remove from oven, score into 2 x 1-inch (5 x 2.5-cm) pieces and cool completely. Break into candy pieces.

YIELD:      60 pieces
EXCHANGE 1 PIECE:   ½ fat
        1/3 bread
CALORIES 1 PIECE:   48

# Fruit Candy Bars

| 1 envelope | unflavored gelatin | 1 envelope |
| ¼ cup | water | 60 mL |
| 1 cup | dried apricots | 250 mL |
| 1 cup | raisins | 250 mL |
| 1 cup | pecans | 250 mL |
| 1 tablespoon | flour | 15 mL |
| 2 tablespoons | orange peel (grated) | 30 mL |
| 1 teaspoon | rum extract | 5 mL |

Sprinkle gelatin over water; allow to soften for 5 minutes. Heat and stir until gelatin is completely dissolved. Combine apricots, raisins, pecans, flour and orange peel in blender or food processor, working until finely chopped. Add to gelatin mixture. Add rum extract and stir to completely blend. Line 8-inch (20-cm) square pan with plastic wrap or waxed paper. Spread fruit mixture evenly into pan, and set aside to cool completely until candy is firm. Turn out onto cutting board, cut into 24 bars and wrap individually.

**YIELD:** 24 bars
**EXCHANGE 1 BAR:** 1 fruit
½ fat
**CALORIES 1 BAR:** 68

# Coconut Macaroons

| 1 cup | evaporated skimmed milk | 250 mL |
| 2 teaspoons | granulated sugar replacement | 10 mL |
| 3 cups | unsweetened coconut (shredded) | 750 mL |

Combine milk and sugar replacement in large bowl, stirring until sugar replacement dissolves. Add coconut and stir until coconut is completely moistened. Drop by teaspoonfuls onto greased cookie sheets, 2 to 3 inches (5 to 7 cm) apart. Bake at 350° F (175° C) for 15 minutes, or until tops are lightly browned. Remove from pan immediately.

**YIELD:** 48 drops
**EXCHANGE 1 DROP:** 1/5 fruit
½ fat
**CALORIES 1 DROP:** 31

# Chocolate Topping

| | | |
|---|---|---|
| 3 cups | skim milk | 750 mL |
| 2 ounces | unsweetened chocolate | 60 g |
| 3 tablespoons | cornstarch | 45 mL |
| ½ cup | sugar replacement | 125 mL |
| 1 teaspoon | salt | 5 mL |
| 2 tablespoons | butter | 30 mL |
| 2 teaspoons | vanilla extract | 10 mL |

Combine skim milk, chocolate, cornstarch, sugar replacement, and salt in saucepan. Bring to a full boil. Boil for 2 to 3 minutes; remove from heat. Add butter and vanilla extract.

**YIELD:**     3 cups (750 mL)
**EXCHANGE 2 TABLESPOONS (30 mL):**   ½ bread
    ½ fat
**CALORIES 2 TABLESPOONS (30 mL):**   35

# Vanilla Gloss

| | | |
|---|---|---|
| ¼ cup | cold water | 60 mL |
| 2 teaspoons | cornstarch | 10 mL |
| Dash | salt | dash |
| ⅓ cup | sugar replacement 90 mL | |
| 1 teaspoon | vanilla extract | 5 mL |

Blend cold water and cornstarch. Pour into small saucepan. Add salt. Boil until clear and thickened. Remove from heat. Add sugar replacement and vanilla extract. Stir to dissolve. Cool.

**YIELD:**   ¼ cup (60 mL)
**EXCHANGE:**   Negligible
**CALORIES:**   Negligible

# FOOD EXCHANGE LISTS

## One starch exchange equals
15 grams carbohydrate,
3 grams protein,
0–1 grams fat, and
80 calories.

## Bread

| | |
|---|---|
| Bagel | 1/2 (1 oz) |
| Bread, reduced-calorie | 2 slices (1 1/2 oz) |
| Bread, white, whole-wheat, pumpernickel, rye | 1 slice (1 oz) |
| Bread sticks, crisp, 4 in. long x 1/2 in. | 2 (2/3 oz) |
| English muffin | 1/2 |
| Hot dog or hamburger bun | 1/2 (1 oz) |
| Pita, 6 in. across | 1/2 |
| Roll, plain, small | 1 (1 oz) |
| Raisin bread, unfrosted | 1 slice (1 oz) |
| Tortilla, corn, 6 in. across | 1 |
| Tortilla, flour, 6 in. across | 1 |
| Waffle, 4 1/2 in. square, reduced-fat | 1 |

## Cereals And Grains

| | |
|---|---|
| Bran cereals | 1/2 cup |
| Bulgur | 1/2 cup |
| Cereals | 1/2 cup |
| Cereals, unsweetened, ready-to-eat | 3/4 cup |
| Cornmeal (dry) | 3 Tbsp |
| Couscous | 1/3 cup |
| Flour (dry) | 3 Tbsp |
| Granola, low-fat | 1/4 cup |
| Grape-Nuts | 1/4 cup |
| Grits | 1/2 cup |
| Kasha | 1/2 cup |
| Millet | 1/4 cup |
| Muesli | 1/4 cup |
| Oats | 1/2 cup |
| Pasta | 1/2 cup |
| Puffed cereal | 1 1/2 cups |
| Rice milk | 1/2 cup |
| Rice, white or brown | 1/3 cup |
| Shredded Wheat | 1/2 cup |
| Sugar-frosted cereal | 1/2 cup |
| Wheat germ | 3 Tbsp |

## One starch exchange equals
**15 grams carbohydrate,
3 grams protein,
0–1 grams fat, and
80 calories.**

## Starchy Vegetables

| | |
|---|---|
| Baked beans | 1/3 cup |
| Corn | 1/2 cup |
| Corn on cob, medium | 1 (5 oz) |
| Mixed vegetables with corn, peas, or pasta | 1 cup |
| Peas, green | 1/2 cup |
| Plantain | 1/2 cup |
| Potato, baked or boiled | 1 small (3 oz) |
| Potato, mashed | 1/2 cup |
| Squash, winter (acorn, butternut, pumpkin) | 1 cup |
| Yam, sweet potato, plain | 1/2 cup |

## Crackers And Snacks

| | |
|---|---|
| Animal crackers | 8 |
| Graham crackers, 2 1/2 in. square | 3 |
| Matzoh | 3/4 oz |
| Melba toast | 4 slices |
| Oyster crackers | 24 |
| Popcorn (popped, no fat added or low-fat microwave) | 3 cups |
| Pretzels | 3/4 oz |
| Rice cakes, 4 in. across | 2 |
| Saltine-type crackers | 6 |
| Snack chips, fat-free (tortilla, potato) | 15–20 (3/4 oz) |
| Whole-wheat crackers, no fat added | 2–5 (3/4 oz) |

## Beans, Peas, And Lentils
**(Count as 1 starch exchange, plus 1 very lean meat exchange.)**

| | |
|---|---|
| Beans and peas (garbanzo, pinto, kidney, white, split, black-eyed) | 1/2 cup |
| Lima beans | 2/3 cup |
| Lentils | 1/2 cup |
| Miso▲ | 3 Tbsp |

▲ = 400 mg or more sodium per exchange.

# One starch exchange equals
## 15 grams carbohydrate,
## 3 grams protein,
## 0–1 grams fat, and
## 80 calories.

## Starchy Foods Prepared With Fat
### (Count as 1 starch exchange, plus 1 fat exchange.)

| | |
|---|---|
| Biscuit, 2 1/2 in. across | 1 |
| Chow mein noodles | 1/2 cup |
| Corn bread, 2 in. cube | 1 (2 oz) |
| Crackers, round butter type | 6 |
| Croutons | 1 cup |
| French-fried potatoes | 16–25 (3 oz) |
| Granola | 1/4 cup |
| Muffin, small | 1 (1 1/2 oz) |
| Pancake, 4 in. across | 2 |
| Popcorn, microwave | 3 cups |
| Sandwich crackers, cheese or peanut butter filling | 3 |
| Stuffing, bread (prepared) | 1/3 cup |
| Taco shell, 6 in. across | 2 |
| Waffle, 4 1/2 in. square | 1 |
| Whole–wheat crackers, fat added | 4–6 (1 oz) |

Starches often swell in cooking, so a small amount of uncooked starch will become a much larger amount of cooked food. The following table shows some of the changes.

| Food (Starch Group) | Uncooked | Cooked |
|---|---|---|
| Oatmeal | 3 Tbsp | 1/2 cup |
| Cream of Wheat | 2 Tbsp | 1/2 cup |
| Grits | 3 Tbsp | 1/2 cup |
| Rice | 2 Tbsp | 1/3 cup |
| Spaghetti | 1/4 cup | 1/2 cup |
| Noodles | 1/3 cup | 1/2 cup |
| Macaroni | 1/4 cup | 1/2 cup |
| Dried beans | 1/4 cup | 1/2 cup |
| Dried peas | 1/4 cup | 1/2 cup |
| Lentils | 3 Tbsp | 1/2 cup |

### Common Measurements

| | |
|---|---|
| 3 tsp = 1 Tbsp | 4 ounces = 1/2 cup |
| 4 Tbsp = 1/4 cup | 8 ounces = 1 cup |
| 5 1/3 Tbsp = 1/3 cup | 1 cup = 1/2 pint |

# One fruit exchange equals
## 15 grams carbohydrate and
## 60 calories.
### The weight includes skin, core, seeds, and rind.

## Fruit

| | |
|---|---|
| Apple, unpeeled, small | 1 (4 oz) |
| Applesauce, unsweetened | 1/2 cup |
| Apples, dried | 4 rings |
| Apricots, fresh | 4 whole (5 1/2 oz) |
| Apricots, dried | 8 halves |
| Apricots, canned | 1/2 cup |
| Banana, small | 1 (4 oz) |
| Blackberries | 3/4 cup |
| Blueberries | 3/4 cup |
| Cantaloupe, small | 1/3 melon (11 oz) or 1 cup cubes |
| Cherries, sweet, fresh | 12 (3 oz) |
| Cherries, sweet, canned | 1/2 cup |
| Dates | 3 |
| Figs, fresh | 1 1/2 large or 2 medium (3 1/2 oz) |
| Figs, dried | 1 1/2 |
| Fruit cocktail | 1/2 cup |
| Grapefruit, large | 1/2 (11 oz) |
| Grapefruit sections, canned | 3/4 cup |
| Grapes, small | 17 (3 oz) |
| Honeydew melon | 1 slice (10 oz) or 1 cup cubes |
| Kiwi | 1 (3 1/2 oz) |
| Mandarin oranges, canned | 3/4 cup |
| Mango, small | 1/2 fruit (5 1/2 oz) or 1/2 cup |
| Nectarine, small | 1 (5 oz) |
| Orange, small | 1 (6 1/2 oz) |
| Papaya | 1/2 fruit (8 oz) or 1 cup cubes |
| Peach, medium, fresh | 1 (6 oz) |
| Peaches, canned | 1/2 cup |
| Pear, large, fresh | 1/2 (4 oz) |
| Pears, canned | 1/2 cup |
| Pineapple, fresh | 3/4 cup |
| Pineapple, canned | 1/2 cup |
| Plums, small | 2 (5 oz) |
| Plums, canned | 1/2 cup |
| Prunes, dried | 3 |
| Raisins | 2 Tbsp |
| Raspberries | 1 cup |
| Strawberries | 1 1/4 cup whole berries |
| Tangerines, small | 2 (8 oz) |
| Watermelon | 1 slice (13 1/2 oz) or 1 1/4 cup cubes |

## Fruit Juice

| | |
|---|---|
| Apple juice/cider | 1/2 cup |
| Cranberry juice cocktail | 1/3 cup |
| Cranberry juice cocktail, reduced-calorie | 1 cup |
| Fruit juice blends, 100% juice | 1/3 cup |
| Grape juice | 1/3 cup |
| Grapefruit juice | 1/2 cup |
| Orange juice | 1/2 cup |
| Pineapple juice | 1/2 cup |
| Prune juice | 1/3 cup |

# One milk exchange equals
12 grams carbohydrate and
8 grams protein.

## Fat-free And Low-fat Milk
(0–3 grams fat per serving)

| | |
|---|---|
| Fat-free milk | 1 cup |
| 1/2% milk | 1 cup |
| 1% milk | 1 cup |
| Fat-free or low-fat buttermilk | 1 cup |
| Evaporated fat-free milk | 1/2 cup |
| Fat-free dry milk | 1/3 cup dry |
| Plain nonfat yogurt | 3/4 cup |
| Nonfat or low-fat fruit-flavored yogurt sweetened with aspartame or with a nonnutritive sweetener | 1 cup |

## Reduced-fat
(5 grams fat per serving)

| | |
|---|---|
| 2% milk | 1 cup |
| Plain low-fat yogurt | 3/4 cup |
| Sweet acidophilus milk | 1 cup |

## Whole Milk
(8 grams fat per serving)

| | |
|---|---|
| Whole milk | 1 cup |
| Evaporated whole milk | 1/2 cup |
| Goat's milk | 1 cup |
| Kefir | 1 cup |

## One exchange equals

**15 grams carbohydrate, or 1 starch, or 1 fruit, or 1 milk.**

| Food | Serving Size | Exchanges Per Serving |
|---|---|---|
| Angel food cake, unfrosted | 1/12th cake | 2 carbohydrates |
| Brownie, small, unfrosted | 2 in. square | 1 carbohydrate, 1 fat |
| Cake, unfrosted | 2 in. square | 1 carbohydrate, 1 fat |
| Cake, frosted | 2 in. square | 2 carbohydrates, 1 fat |
| Cookie, fat-free | 2 small | 1 carbohydrate |
| Cookie or sandwich cookie with creme filling | 2 small | 1 carbohydrate, 1 fat |
| Cranberry sauce, jellied | 1/4 cup | 1 1/2 carbohydrates |
| Cupcake, frosted | 1 small | 2 carbohydrates, 1 fat |
| Doughnut, plain cake | 1 medium (1 1/2 oz) | 1 1/2 carbohydrates, 2 fats |
| Doughnut, glazed | 3 3/4 in. across (2 oz) | 2 carbohydrates, 2 fats |
| Fruit juice bars, frozen, 100% juice | 1 bar (3 oz) | 1 carbohydrate |
| Fruit snacks, chewy (pureed fruit concentrate) | 1 roll (3/4 oz) | 1 carbohydrate |
| Fruit spreads, 100% fruit | 1 Tbsp | 1 carbohydrate |
| Gelatin, regular | 1/2 cup | 1 carbohydrate |
| Gingersnaps | 3 | 1 carbohydrate |
| Granola bar | 1 bar | 1 carbohydrate, 1 fat |
| Granola bar, fat-free | 1 bar | 2 carbohydrates |

# One exchange equals

15 grams carbohydrate, or 1 starch, or 1 fruit, or 1 milk.

| Food | Serving Size | Exchanges Per Serving |
|---|---|---|
| Honey | 1 Tbsp | 1 carbohydrate |
| Hummus | 1/3 cup | 1 carbohydrate, 1 fat |
| Ice cream | 1/2 cup | 1 carbohydrate, 2 fats |
| Ice cream, light | 1/2 cup | 1 carbohydrate, 1 fat |
| Ice cream, fat-free, no sugar added | 1/2 cup | 1 carbohydrate |
| Jam or jelly, regular | 1 Tbsp | 1 carbohydrate |
| Milk, chocolate, whole | 1 cup | 2 carbohydrates, 1 fat |
| Pie, fruit, 2 crusts | 1/6 pie | 3 carbohydrates, 2 fats |
| Pie, pumpkin or custard | 1/8 pie | 2 carbohydrates, 2 fats |
| Potato chips | 12–18 (1 oz) | 1 carbohydrate, 2 fats |
| Pudding, regular (made with low-fat milk) | 1/2 cup | 2 carbohydrates |
| Pudding, sugar-free (made with low-fat milk) | 1/2 cup | 1 carbohydrate |
| Salad dressing, fat-free ◀ | 1/4 cup | 1 carbohydrate |
| Sherbet, sorbet | 1/2 cup | 2 carbohydrates |
| Spaghetti or pasta sauce, canned ◀ | 1/2 cup | 1 carbohydrate, 1 fat |
| Sugar | 1 Tbsp | 1 carbohydrate |
| Sweet roll or Danish | 1 (2 1/2 oz) | 2 1/2 carbohydrates, 2 fats |
| Syrup, light | 2 Tbsp | 1 carbohydrate |
| Syrup, regular | 1 Tbsp | 1 carbohydrate |
| Syrup, regular | 1/4 cup | 4 carbohydrates |
| Tortilla chips | 6–12 (1 oz) | 1 carbohydrate, 2 fats |
| Vanilla wafers | 5 | 1 carbohydrate, 1 fat |
| Yogurt, frozen, low-fat, fat-free | 1/3 cup | 1 carbohydrate, 0–1 fat |
| Yogurt, frozen, fat-free, no sugar added | 1/2 cup | 1 carbohydrate |
| Yogurt, low-fat with fruit | 1 cup | 3 carbohydrates, 0–1 fat |

◀ = 400 mg or more of sodium per exchange.

## One vegetable exchange equals
5 grams carbohydrate,
2 grams protein,
0 grams fat, and
25 calories.

Artichoke
Artichoke hearts
Asparagus
Beans (green, wax, Italian)
Bean sprouts
Beets
Broccoli
Brussels sprouts
Cabbage
Carrots
Cauliflower
Celery
Cucumber
Eggplant
Green onions or scallions
Greens (collard, kale, mustard, turnip)
Kohlrabi
Leeks
Mixed vegetables (without corn, peas, or pasta)
Mushrooms
Okra
Onions

Pea pods
Peppers (all varieties)
Radishes
Salad greens (endive, escarole, lettuce, romaine, spinach)
Sauerkraut ◢
Spinach
Summer squash
Tomato
Tomatoes, canned
Tomato sauce ◢
Tomato/vegetable juice ◢
Turnips
Water chestnuts
Watercress
Zucchini

◢ = 400 mg or more sodium per exchange.

# Very Lean Meat And Substitutes List
**One exchange equals 0 grams carbohydrate, 7 grams protein, 0-1 grams fat, and 35 calories.**

- One very lean meat exchange is equal to any one of the following items.

**Poultry:** Chicken or turkey (white meat, no skin), Cornish hen (no skin) ......1 oz

**Fish:** Fresh or frozen cod, flounder, haddock, halibut, trout; tuna fresh or canned in water ......1 oz

**Shellfish:** Clams, crab, lobster, scallops, shrimp, imitation shellfish......1 oz

**Game:** Duck or pheasant (no skin), venison, buffalo, ostrich......1 oz

**Cheese with 1 gram or less fat per ounce:**
Nonfat or low-fat cottage cheese ......1/4 cup
Fat-free cheese ......1 oz

**Other:** Processed sandwich meats with 1 gram or less fat per ounce, such as deli thin, shaved meats, chipped beef▲, turkey ham......1 oz
Egg whites......2
Egg substitutes, plain ......1/4 cup
Hot dogs with 1 gram or less fat per ounce▲......1 oz
Kidney (high in cholesterol)......1 oz
Sausage with 1 gram or less fat per ounce......1 oz

- Count as one very lean meat and one starch exchange.

Beans, peas, lentils (cooked) ......1/2 cup

▲ = 400 mg or more sodium per exchange.

# Lean Meat And Substitutes List
**One exchange equals 0 grams carbohydrate, 7 grams protein, 3 grams fat, and 55 calories.**

- One lean meat exchange is equal to any one of the following items.

**Beef:** USDA Select or Choice grades of lean beef trimmed of fat, such as round, sirloin, and flank steak; tenderloin; roast (rib, chuck, rump); steak (T-bone, porterhouse, cubed), ground round......1 oz

**Pork:** Lean pork, such as fresh ham; canned, cured, or boiled ham; Canadian bacon▲; tenderloin, center loin chop......1 oz

**Lamb:** Roast, chop, leg......1 oz

**Veal:** Lean chop, roast......1 oz

**Poultry:** Chicken, turkey (dark meat, no skin), chicken (white meat, with skin), domestic duck or goose (well-drained of fat, no skin) ......1 oz

**Fish:**
Herring (uncreamed or smoked)......1 oz
Oysters......6 medium
Salmon (fresh or canned), catfish......1 oz
Sardines (canned) ......2 medium
Tuna (canned in oil, drained) ......1 oz

**Game:** Goose (no skin), rabbit ......1 oz

**Cheese:**
4.5%-fat cottage cheese......1/4 cup
Grated Parmesan......2 Tbsp
Cheeses with 3 grams or less fat per ounce ......1 oz

**Other:**
Hot dogs with 3 grams or less fat per ounce▲ ......1 1/2 oz
Processed sandwich meat with 3 grams or less fat per ounce, such as turkey pastrami or kielbasa......1 oz
Liver, heart (high in cholesterol) ......1 oz

## Medium-Fat Meat And Substitutes List
### One exchange equals 0 grams carbohydrate, 7 grams protein, 5 grams fat, and 75 calories.

● One medium-fat meat exchange is equal to any one of the following items.

**Beef:** Most beef products fall into this category (ground beef, meatloaf, corned beef, short ribs, Prime grades of meat trimmed of fat, such as prime rib) ....... 1 oz

**Pork:** Top loin, chop, Boston butt, cutlet. ................ 1 oz

**Lamb:** Rib roast, ground ................................... 1 oz

**Veal:** Cutlet (ground or cubed, unbreaded) .............. 1 oz

**Poultry:** Chicken (dark meat, with skin), ground turkey or ground chicken, fried chicken (with skin) ........... 1 oz

**Fish:** Any fried fish product. ............................ 1 oz

**Cheese:** With 5 grams or less fat per ounce

Feta. ....................................................... 1 oz
Mozzarella ................................................. 1 oz
Ricotta ................................................. 1/4 cup (2 oz)

**Other:**
Egg (high in cholesterol, limit to 3 per week) ........... 1
Sausage with 5 grams or less fat per ounce ............... 1 oz
Soy milk ................................................. 1 cup
Tempeh ................................................. 1/4 cup
Tofu ................................................. 4 oz or 1/2 cup

▰ = 400 mg or more sodium per exchange.

## High-Fat Meat And Substitutes List
### One exchange equals 0 grams carbohydrate, 7 grams protein, 8 grams fat, and 100 calories.

Remember these items are high in saturated fat, cholesterol, and calories and may raise blood cholesterol levels if eaten on a regular basis.

● One high-fat meat exchange is equal to any one of the following items.

**Pork:** Spareribs, ground pork, pork sausage ............ 1 oz

**Cheese:** All regular cheeses, such as American▰, cheddar, Monterey Jack, Swiss ....................... 1 oz

**Other:** Processed sandwich meats with 8 grams or less fat per ounce, such as bologna, pimento loaf, salami ............................................. 1 oz
Sausage, such as bratwurst, Italian, knockwurst, Polish, smoked ......................... 1 oz
Hot dog (turkey or chicken)▰ .................... 1 (10/lb)
Bacon ................................... 3 slices (20 slices/lb)

● Count as one high-fat meat plus one fat exchange.

Hot dog (beef, pork, or combination)▰ ........... 1 (10/lb)

● Count as one high-fat meat plus two fat exchanges.

Peanut butter (contains unsaturated fat) ............. 2 Tbsp

## Monounsaturated Fats List
**One fat exchange equals 5 grams fat and 45 calories.**

| | |
|---|---|
| Avocado, medium | 1/8 (1 oz) |
| Oil (canola, olive, peanut) | 1 tsp |
| Olives: ripe (black)◀ | 8 large |
| green, stuffed◀ | 10 large |
| Nuts | |
| almonds, cashews | 6 nuts |
| mixed (50% peanuts) | 6 nuts |
| peanuts | 10 nuts |
| pecans | 4 halves |
| Peanut butter, smooth or crunchy | 2 tsp |
| Sesame seeds | 1 Tbsp |
| Tahini paste | 2 tsp |

## Polyunsaturated Fats List
**One fat exchange equals 5 grams fat and 45 calories.**

| | |
|---|---|
| Margarine: stick, tub, or squeeze | 1 tsp |
| lower-fat (30% to 50% vegetable oil) | 1 Tbsp |
| Mayonnaise: regular | 1 tsp |
| reduced-fat | 1 Tbsp |
| Nuts, walnuts, English | 4 halves |
| Oil (corn, safflower, soybean) | 1 tsp |
| Salad dressing: regular◀ | 1 Tbsp |
| reduced-fat | 2 Tbsp |
| Miracle Whip Salad Dressing®: regular | 2 tsp |
| reduced-fat | 1 Tbsp |
| Seeds: pumpkin, sunflower | 1 Tbsp |

◀ = 400 mg or more sodium per exchange.

## Saturated Fats List*
**One fat exchange equals 5 grams of fat and 45 calories.**

| | |
|---|---|
| Bacon, cooked | 1 slice (20 slices/lb) |
| Bacon, grease | 1 tsp |
| Butter: stick | 1 tsp |
| whipped | 2 tsp |
| reduced-fat | 1 Tbsp |
| Chitterlings, boiled | 2 Tbsp (1/2 oz) |
| Coconut, sweetened, shredded | 2 Tbsp |
| Cream, half and half | 2 Tbsp |
| Cream cheese: regular | 1 Tbsp (1/2 oz) |
| reduced-fat | 2 Tbsp (1 oz) |
| Fatback or salt pork, see below† | |
| Shortening or lard | 1 tsp |
| Sour cream: regular | 2 Tbsp |
| reduced-fat | 3 Tbsp |

†Use a piece 1 in. x 1 in. x 1/4 in. if you plan to eat the fatback cooked with vegetables. Use a piece 2 in. x 1 in. x 1/2 in. when eating only the vegetables with the fatback removed.

*Saturated fats can raise blood cholesterol levels.

# Free Foods List

A *free food* is any food or drink that contains less than 20 calories or less than 5 grams of carbohydrate per serving. Foods with a serving size listed should be limited to three servings per day. Be sure to spread them out throughout the day. If you eat all three servings at one time, it could affect your blood glucose level. Foods listed without a serving size can be eaten as often as you like.

## Fat-free Or Reduced-fat Foods

| | |
|---|---|
| Cream cheese, fat-free | 1 Tbsp |
| Creamers, nondairy, liquid | 1 Tbsp |
| Creamers, nondairy, powdered | 2 tsp |
| Mayonnaise, fat-free | 1 Tbsp |
| Mayonnaise, reduced-fat | 1 tsp |
| Margarine, fat-free | 4 Tbsp |
| Margarine, reduced-fat | 1 tsp |
| Miracle Whip®, nonfat | 1 Tbsp |
| Miracle Whip®, reduced-fat | 1 tsp |
| Nonstick cooking spray | |
| Salad dressing, fat-free | 1 Tbsp |
| Salad dressing, fat-free, Italian | 2 Tbsp |
| Salsa | 1/4 cup |
| Sour cream, fat-free, reduced-fat | 1 Tbsp |
| Whipped topping, regular or light | 2 Tbsp |

## Sugar-free Or Low-sugar Foods

| | |
|---|---|
| Candy, hard, sugar-free | 1 candy |
| Gelatin dessert, sugar-free | |
| Gelatin, unflavored | |
| Gum, sugar-free | |
| Jam or jelly, low-sugar or light | 2 tsp |
| Sugar substitutes[†] | |
| Syrup, sugar-free | 2 Tbsp |

[†]Sugar substitutes, alternatives, or replacements that are approved by the Food and Drug Administration (FDA) are safe to use. Common brand names include:

Equal® (aspartame)
Sprinkle Sweet® (saccharin)
Sweet One® (acesulfame K)
Sweet-10® (saccharin)
Sugar Twin® (saccharin)
Sweet 'n Low® (saccharin)

## Drinks

Bouillon, broth, consommé ✎
Bouillon or broth, low-sodium
Carbonated or mineral water
Club soda
Cocoa powder, unsweetened . . . . . . . . . . . . . . . . . . . . . . . 1 Tbsp
Coffee
Diet soft drinks, sugar-free
Drink mixes, sugar-free
Tea
Tonic water, sugar-free

## Condiments

Catsup . . . . . . . . . . . . . . . . . . . . . . . . . . . . . . . . . . . . . . . . 1 Tbsp
Horseradish
Lemon juice
Lime juice
Mustard
Pickles, dill ✎ . . . . . . . . . . . . . . . . . . . . . . . . . . . . . . 1 1/2 large
Soy sauce, regular or light ✎
Taco sauce . . . . . . . . . . . . . . . . . . . . . . . . . . . . . . . . . . . . 1 Tbsp
Vinegar

## Seasonings

Be careful with seasonings that contain sodium or are salts, such as garlic or celery salt, and lemon pepper.

Flavoring extracts
Garlic
Herbs, fresh or dried
Pimento
Spices
Tabasco® or hot pepper sauce
Wine, used in cooking
Worcestershire sauce

✎ = 400 mg or more of sodium per exchange.

# Combination Foods List

Many of the foods we eat are mixed together in various combinations. These combination foods do not fit into any one exchange list. Often it is hard to tell what is in a casserole dish or prepared food item. This is a list of exchanges for some typical combination foods. This list will help you fit these foods into your meal plan. Ask your dietitian for information about any other combination foods you would like to eat.

| Food | Serving Size | Exchanges Per Serving |
|---|---|---|
| **Entrees** | | |
| Tuna noodle casserole, lasagna, spaghetti with meatballs, chili with beans, macaroni and cheese◢ | 1 cup (8 oz) | 2 carbohydrates, 2 medium-fat meats |
| Chow mein (without noodles or rice)◢ | 2 cups (16 oz) | 1 carbohydrate, 2 lean meats |
| Pizza, cheese, thin crust◢ | 1/4 of 10 in. (5 oz) | 2 carbohydrates, 2 medium-fat meats, 1 fat |
| Pizza, meat topping, thin crust◢ | 1/4 of 10 in. (5 oz) | 2 carbohydrates, 2 medium-fat meats, 2 fats |
| Pot pie◢ | 1 (7 oz) | 2 carbohydrates, 1 medium-fat meat, 4 fats |
| **Frozen entrees** | | |
| Salisbury steak with gravy, mashed potato◢ | 1 (11 oz) | 2 carbohydrates, 3 medium-fat meats, 3–4 fats |
| Turkey with gravy, mashed potato, dressing◢ | 1 (11 oz) | 2 carbohydrates, 2 medium-fat meats, 2 fats |
| Entree with less than 300 calories◢ | 1 (8 oz) | 2 carbohydrates, 3 lean meats |
| **Soups** | | |
| Bean◢ | 1 cup | 1 carbohydrate, 1 very lean meat |
| Cream (made with water)◢ | 1 cup (8 oz) | 1 carbohydrate, 1 fat |
| Split pea (made with water)◢ | 1/2 cup (4 oz) | 1 carbohydrate |
| Tomato (made with water)◢ | 1 cup (8 oz) | 1 carbohydrate |
| Vegetable beef, chicken noodle, or other broth-type◢ | 1 cup (8 oz) | 1 carbohydrate |

◢ = 400 mg or more sodium per exchange.

**239**

# Bread

| | Product | Amount | Calories | Exchange |
|---|---|---|---|---|
| Best Foods, CPC International | Argo Cornstarch | 2T. (30 ml) | 70 | 1 bread |
| | Duryea's Cornstarch | 2T. (30 ml) | 70 | 1 bread |
| | Kingsford Cornstarch | 2T. (30 ml) | 70 | 1 bread |
| | Presto Self-Rising Cake Flour | 2 ½ T. (35 mL) | 60 | 1 bread |
| Creamette Co. | Egg Noodles (cooked) | 1 c. (250 mL) | 220 | 3 bread |
| | Macaroni and Cheese Dinner (cooked) | 1 c. (250 mL) | 240 | 3 bread 2 fat |
| | Pasta Misc. (cooked) | 1 c. | 210 | 3 bread |
| General Foods | Stove Top Stuffing Mixes | ½ c. (125 mL) | 180 | 1½ bread 2 fat |
| General Mills | Bisquick | 2 oz. (60 g) | 240 | 2½ bread 1½ fat |
| | POTATOES: 1 portion, prepared as directed | | | |
| | Au Gratin | | 150 | 1½ bread 1 fat |
| | Creamed | | 160 | 1½ bread 1 fat |
| | Hash Browns with Onions | | 150 | 1½ bread 1 fat |
| | Julienne | | 130 | 1 bread 1 fat |
| | Potato Buds | | 130 | 1 bread 1 fat |
| | Scalloped | | 150 | 1½ bread 1 fat |
| | Sour Cream 'n Chive | | 140 | 1 bread 1 fat |

| | Product | Amount | Calories | Exchange |
|---|---|---|---|---|
| Pillsbury | PIE CRUSTS: Prepared According to basic recipe | | | |
| | Mix or Stick | ⅙ crust | 145 | 1 bread 1 fat |
| | OTHER BREADS: Prepared according to basic recipe | | | |
| | Hot Roll Mix | 1 roll | 95 | 1 bread ½ fat |
| | Hotloaf | 1 slice | 90 | 1 bread ½ fat |
| | HUNGRY JACK BISCUITS | | | |
| | Butter Tastin' | 1 biscuits | 190 | 1½ bread 2 fat |
| | Flaky | 2 biscuits | 180 | 1½ bread 2 fat |
| | Flaky Buttermilk | 2 biscuits | 180 | 1½ bread 2 fat |
| | Fluffy Buttermilk | 2 biscuits | 190 | 1½ bread 2 fat |
| | PILLSBURY BISCUITS | | | |
| | Buttermilk | 2 biscuits | 110 | 1½ bread |
| | Country Style | 2 biscuits | 110 | 1½ bread |
| | Flaky Tenderflake Buttermilk Dinner | 2 biscuits | 120 | 1 bread 2 fat |
| | Tenderflake Baking Powder Dinner | 2 biscuits | 120 | 1 bread 1 fat |
| | HUNGRY JACK POTATOES: Prepared according to basic recipe | | | |
| | Mashed Potato Flakes | ½ c. (125 mL) | 140 | 1 bread 1 ½ fat |
| | HUNGRY JACK PANCAKE & WAFFLE MIXES: 1 pancake, 4 in. (10 cm) prepared According to basic recipe | | | |
| | Blueberry | | 113 | 1 bread 1 fat |
| | Buttermilk | | 80 | ½ bread 1 fat |

| | Product | Amount | Calories | Exchange |
|---|---|---|---|---|
| Pillsbury | **DINNER ROLLS** | | | |
| | Oven Lovin' | 2 rolls | 110 | 1 bread ½ fat |
| | Pillsbury Crescent | 2 rolls | 190 | 1½ bread 2 fat |
| | **MUFFINS** Apple, Cinnamon, Bran, Or Corn | 1 muffin | 120 | 1 bread 1 fat |
| | **WIENER WRAPS** Cheese | 1 wrap | 70 | ½ bread ½ fat |
| | Plain | 1 wrap | 60 | ½ bread ½ fat |

## MEATS

| | Product | Amount | Calories | Exchange |
|---|---|---|---|---|
| Hormel | Coarse-Ground Bologna | 2 oz. | 150 | 1 high-fat meat ½ vegetable |
| | Chopped Ham | 1 oz. | 70 | 1 lean meat ½ fat |
| | Deviled Ham | 1 oz. | 70 | ½ lean meat |
| | Kolbase Polish Sausage | 3 oz. | 70 | 2 high-fat meat 1 fat |
| | Meat or Beef Wieners, | 1 | 140 | 1 high-fat meat |
| | Spam | 3 oz. | 260 | 1½ medium-fat meat ½ vegetable |
| | Tender Chunk Chicken | 3 oz. | 110 | 2 lean meat |
| | Tender Chunk Ham | 3 oz. | 140 | 2 medium-fat meat |

| | Product | Amount | Calories | Exchange |
|---|---|---|---|---|
| Hormel | Tender Chunk Turkey | 3 oz.<br>(90 g) | 90 | 2 lean meat |
| Oscar Mayer | Beef Bologna | 1 slice | 75 | ½ meat<br>1 fat |
| | Beef Cotto Salami | 1 slice | 50 | ½ meat<br>½ fat |
| | Beef Franks | 1 | 140 | ½ meat<br>2 fat |
| | Braunschweiger | 1 slice | 70 | ½ meat<br>1 fat |
| | Chopped Ham | 1 slice | 65 | ½ meat<br>½ fat |
| | Cooked Ham | 1 slice | 30 | ½ meat |
| | Hard Salami | 1 slice | 35 | ¼ meat<br>½ fat |
| | Honey Loaf | 1 slice | 35 | ½ meat |
| | Jubilee Canned Ham | 1 oz.<br>(30 g) | 35 | ½ meat |
| | Little Friers Pork Sausage | 1 | 65 | ½ meat<br>1 fat |
| | New England Brand Sausage | 1 | 35 | ½ meat |
| | Sandwich Spread | 1 oz.<br>(30 g) | 60 | ½ meat<br>½ fat |

## Casseroles and One-Dish Meals

| | Product | Amount | Calories | Exchange |
|---|---|---|---|---|
| Franco-American | Beef Ravioli in Meat Sauce | 7 ½ oz.<br>(225 g) | 220 | 1 vegetable<br>2 bread<br>1 lean meat |
| | Elbow Macaroni & Cheese | 7 ¼ oz.<br>(220 g) | 180 | 2 bread<br>1 fat |
| | Rotini in Tomato Sauce | 7 ½ oz.<br>(225 g) | 200 | 1 vegetable<br>1 fat |
| | Spaghetti in Meat Sauce | 7 ¾ oz.<br>(230 g) | 220 | 1 vegetable<br>1 bread<br>1 lean meat<br>1 fat |

| | Product | Amount | Calories | Exchange |
|---|---|---|---|---|
| Franco-American | Spaghetti-O's in Tomato & Cheese Sauce | 7 ½ oz. (225 g) | 160 | 2 bread |
| General Mills | HAMBURGER HELPER: 1 portion, prepared as directed | | | |
| | Beef Noodle | | 320 | 2 bread 2 medium-fat meat ½ fat |
| | Cheeseburger Macaroni | | 360 | 1½ bread ½ milk 2 medium-fat meat 1 fat |
| | Lasagne | | 330 | 2 bread 2 medium-fat meat ½ fat |
| | Hamburger Pizza Dish | | 340 | 2 bread 2 medium-fat meat ½ fat |
| | Hamburger Stew | | 290 | 1 bread 1 vegetable 2 medium-fat meat 1 fat |
| | Potato Stroganoff | | 330 | 2 bread 2 medium-fat meat ½ fat |
| | Rice Oriental | 8-oz. pkg. (240-g pkg.) | 340 | 2 bread 2 medium-fat meat ½ fat |
| | Spaghetti | | 330 | 2 bread 2 medium-fat meat |

| Product | Amount | Calories | Exchange |
|---|---|---|---|
| **General Mills** | | | ½ fat |
| TUNA HELPER: | | | |
| 1 portion, prepared as directed | | | |
| Country Dumplings 'n Tuna | | 230 | 2 bread |
| | | | 1 lean meat |
| | | | ½ fat |
| Creamy Noodles 'n Tuna | | 280 | 2 bread |
| | | | 1 lean meat |
| | | | 1½ fat |
| Noodles, Cheese Sauce 'n Tuna | | 230 | 1½ bread |
| | | | ½ milk |
| | | | 1 lean meat |
| | | | ½ fat |
| CASSEROLES AND SIDE DISHES: | | | |
| 1 portion, prepared as directed | | | |
| Macaroni & Cheese | | 310 | 2 bread |
| | | | ½ milk |
| | | | 3 fat |
| Noodles Romanoff | | 230 | 1 bread |
| | | | ½ milk |
| | | | 2 ½ fat |
| Noodles Stroganoff | | 230 | 1½ bread |
| | | | ½ milk |
| | | | 2 fat |
| **Hormel** | SHORT ORDERS: | | |
| | 7½-oz. (225-g) can | | |
| Beans 'n Wieners | | 290 | 1 high-fat meat |
| | | | 1 fat |
| | | | 2 bread |
| Beef Goulash | | 230 | 2 medium-fat meat |
| | | | 1 bread |
| Chili with Beans | | 300 | 2 high-fat meat |
| | | | 1½ bread |
| Lasagne | | 260 | 1 high-fat meat |

| Product | Amount | Calories | Exchange |
|---------|--------|----------|----------|
| | | | 1½ fat |
| | | | 1½ bread |
| **Hormel** Spaghetti'n Beef | | 2401 | high-fat meat |
| | | | 1 fat |
| | | | 1½ bread |
| **Swanson** FROZEN MEAT PIES: 1 complete pie | | | |
| Beef | 8 oz. (240 g) | 430 | 3 bread 1 lean meat 4 fat |
| Chicken and Turkey | 8 oz. (240 g) | 450 | 3 bread 1 lean meat 4 fat |
| Macaroni and Cheese | 7 oz. (210 g) | 230 | 2 bread 1 lean meat 1 fat |
| HUNGRY MAN MEAT PIES: | | | |
| Beef | 16 oz. (480 g) | 770 | 1 vegetable 4 bread 3 lean meat 7 fat |
| Chicken | 16 oz. (480 g) | 780 | 1 vegetable 4 bread 3 lean meat 7 fat |
| Turkey | 16 oz. (480 g) | 790 | 1 vegetable 4 bread 3 lean meat 7 fat |
| ENTREES: 1 complete entrée | | | |
| Chicken Nibbles with French Fries | 6 oz. (180 g) | 370 | 2 bread 2 lean meat 3 fat |
| Fried Chicken with Whipped Potatoes | 7oz. (210 g) | 360 | 2 bread 2 lean meat 2 fat |
| Gravy & Sliced Beef with Whipped Potatoes | 8 oz. (240 g) | 190 | 1½ bread 1 lean meat |

| Product | Amount | Calories | Exchange |
|---|---|---|---|
| **Swanson** | | | 1 fat |
| | | | 3 fat |
| Spaghetti with Breaded Veal | 8¼ oz. | 290 | 2 bread |
| | (250 g) | | 1 lean meat |
| | | | 2 fat |
| Turkey/Gravy/Dressing with Whipped Potatoes | 8 ¾ oz | 260 | 2 bread |
| | (280 g) | | 2 lean meat |
| HUNGRY MAN ENTREES: | | | |
| Barbecue Chicken with Whipped Potato | 12 oz. (360 g) | 550 | 3 bread |
| | | | 4 lean meat |
| | | | 3 fat |
| Sliced Beef with Whipped Potatoes | 12 ¼ oz. (370 g) | 330 | 1½ bread |
| | | | 4 lean meat |
| Turkey/Gravy/Dressing with Whipped Potatoes | 13 ¼ oz. (400 g) | 380 | 2 bread |
| | | | 4 lean meat |

## Sandwiches and Snacks

| Product | Amount | Calories | Exchange |
|---|---|---|---|
| Best Foods, CPC International | | | |
| Skippy Dry-Roasted Peanuts, Cashews, Mixed Nuts | 1 oz. | 165 | 1 medium-fat meat |
| | (30 g) | | 2 fat |
| General Mills — Beef Jerky | 1 strip | 25 | ½ lean meat |
| Kraft Pizza — Cheese | ¼ pizza | 250 | 2 ½ bread |
| | | | 1 medium-fat meat |
| Sausage | ¼ pizza | 280 | 2½ bread |
| | | | 1 fat |
| | | | 1 medium-fat meat |
| Ore-Ida Foods — Onion Ringers | 2 oz. (60 g) | 160 | 1 bread |
| | | | 2 fat |
| La Pizzeria Pizza, Pepperoni | 5.3 oz. (160 g) | 330 | 3 bread |
| | | | 1 fat |
| | | | 2 medium-fat meat |

| | Product | Amount | Calories | Exchange |
|---|---|---|---|---|
| Ore-Ida Foods | La Pizzeria Pizza, Thick Crust, Cheese | 6.2 oz. (180 g) | 410 | 3 bread<br>1 fat<br>2 medium-fat meat |
| Planters | OIL-ROASTED NUTS:<br>Cashews | 1 oz. (30 g) | 180 | 1 bread<br>1 high-fat meat |
| | Mixed (with peanuts) | 1 oz. (30 g) | 185 | 1 fruit or ½ bread<br>1 high-fat meat |
| | Mixed (without peanuts) | 1 oz. (30 g) | 185 | 1 fruit or ½ bread<br>1 high-fat meat |
| | Peanuts | ¾ oz. | 130 | 1 high-fat meat |
| | DRY ROASTED NUTS:<br>Almonds | 1 oz. (30 g) | 185 | 1 fruit or ½ bread<br>1 high-fat meat |
| | Cashews | 1oz (30 g). | 180 | 1 fruit or ½ bread<br>1 high-fat meat |
| | Mixed | 1oz.(30 g) | 175 | 1 fruit or ½ bread<br>1 high-fat meat |
| | Peanuts | 1oz (30 g). | 170 | 1 fruit or ½ bread<br>1 high-fat meat |

# Fast-Food Items

| | Fast-Food Items | Amount | Calories | Exchange |
|---|---|---|---|---|
| Burger King | Hamburger | 1 | 240 | 1½ bread<br>1 medium-fat meat<br>1 fat |
| | Double-Meat Hamburger | 1 | 370 | 1½ bread<br>3 medium-fat meat<br>1 fat |
| | Cheeseburger | 1 | 310 | 2 bread<br>2 medium-fat meat<br>1 fat |
| | Double Meat Cheesburger Hamburger | 1 | 420 | 2 bread<br>3 medium-fat meat<br>1½ fat |
| | Whopper, Jr. | 1 | 300 | 2 bread<br>1 medium-fat meat<br>2 fat |
| | Whopper, Jr. with Cheese | 1 | 350 | 2 bread<br>2 medium-fat meat<br>2 fat |
| | Double Meat Whopper, Jr. | 1 | 410 | 2 bread<br>2 medium-fat meat<br>3 fat |
| | Double Meat Whopper, Jr. With Cheese | 1 | 460 | 2 bread<br>3 medium-fat meat<br>2½ fat |
| | Whopper | 1 | 650 | 3½ bread<br>3 medium-fat meat<br>4 ½ fat |
| | Whopper with Cheese | 1 | 760 | 3½ bread |

| Fast-Food Items | Amount | Calories | Exchange |
|---|---|---|---|
| **Burger King** | | | 4 medium-fat meat 5½ fat |
| French Fries (small) | 1 | 200 | 2 bread 2 fat |
| French Fries (large) | 1 | 320 | 3 bread 3 fat |
| Onion Rings (small) | 1 | 150 | 1 bread 1 vegetable 1½ fat |
| Onion Rings (large) | 1 | 220 | 2 bread 1 vegetable 2 fat |
| **Kentucky Fried Chicken** | | | |
| Fried Chicken, mashed potato, coleslaw, rolls | | | |
| Original 3-piece dinner | | 830 | 4 bread 6 meat 2½ fat |
| Crispy 3-piece dinner | | 1070 | 5 bread 6 meat 6½ fat |
| Original 2-piece dinner | | 595 | 3½ bread 2 meat 1½ fat |
| Crispy 2-piece dinner | | 665 | 3 bread 4½ meat 3½ fat |
| **McDonalds** Hamburger | 1 | 260 | 1½ bread 1 meat 1½ fat |
| Double Hamburger | 1 | 350 | 2 bread 2 meat 1 fat |
| Quarter Pounder | 1 | 420 | 2½ bread 3 meat 1 fat |
| Big Mac | 1 | 550 | 3 bread 2 meat |

| Fast-Food Items | Amount | Calories | Exchange |
|---|---|---|---|
| McDonalds | | | 4 fat |
| French Fries | 1 | 180 | 1½ bread |
| | | | 2 fat |
| Chocolate Milk Shake | 1 | 315 | 3½ bread |
| | | | 1½ fat |
| Pizza Hut Cheese Pizza | | | |
| Thick Crust, individual | 1 | 1030 | 9½ bread |
| | | | 7½ meat |
| Thin Crust, individual | 1 | 1005 | 8 ½ bread |
| | | | 6 meat |
| Thick Crust, 13 in. | half (32.5 cm) | 900 | 7½ bread |
| | | | 7 meat |
| Thin Crust, 13 in. | half (32.5 cm) | 850 | 7 bread |
| | | | 5 meat |
| Totino's PARTY PIZZAS. | | | |
| Cheese, 13 oz (369 g) | half | 440 | 3 bread |
| | | | 1 vegetable |
| | | | 2 medium-fat meat |
| | | | 1 fat |
| Pepperoni, 13 oz (369 g) | half | 460 | 3 bread |
| | | | 1 vegetable |
| | | | 2 medium-fat meat |
| | | | 1½ fat |
| Sausage, 13 oz (383 g) | half | 470 | 3 bread |
| | | | 1 vegetable |
| | | | 2 medium-fat meat |
| | | | 1½ fat |

## Sauces and Salad Dressings

| Product | Amount | Calories | Exchange |
|---|---|---|---|
| Best Foods, CPC International Hellman's French | 1 T. (15 mL) | 60 | 1 fat |

| | Product | Amount | Calories | Exchange |
|---|---|---|---|---|
| Best Foods, CPC International | Hellman's Real Mayonaise | 1 t. (5 mL) | 35 | 1 fat |
| | Hellman's Sandwich Spread | 2t. (10 mL) | 40 | 1 fat |
| | Hellman's Spin Blend | 1t. (10 mL) | 40 | 1 fat |
| | Hellman's Tartar Sauce | 2t. (15 mL) | 50 | 1 fat |
| Cambell's | Beef Gravy | 2 oz. (60 g) | 30 | 1 fat |
| | Brown Gravy with Onions | 2 oz. (60 g) | 25 | 1 fat |
| | Chicken Gravy | 2 oz. (60 g) | 50 | 1 fat |
| | Chicken Giblet Gravy | 2 oz. (60 g) | 35 | 1 fat |
| | Mushroom Gravy | 2 oz (60 g) | 35 | 1 fat |
| Chiffon Products | Lo-Cal French | 1 T. (15 mL) | 25 | ½ fat |
| | Lo-Cal Italian | 1 T. (15 mL) | 40 | 1 fat |
| | Seven Seas Salad Dressing | 1 T. (15 mL) | 70 | 1½ fat |
| Kraft Products | Miracle Whip | 1 T. (15 mL) | 70 | 1½ fat |
| | Real Mayonaise | 1 T. (15 mL) | 10 | 2 fat |
| Pillsbury | Brown or Homestyle Gravy | ½ c. (125 mL) | 30 | ½ bread |
| | Chicken Gravy | ½ c. | 30 | ½ bread |

# INDEX